CAREGIVER'S HANDBOOK

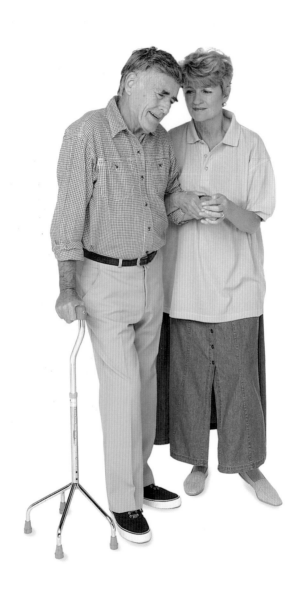

VISITING NURSE ASSOCIATIONS OF AMERICA

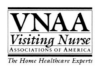

VNAA
Visiting Nurse
ASSOCIATIONS OF AMERICA
The Home Healthcare Experts

CAREGIVER'S HANDBOOK

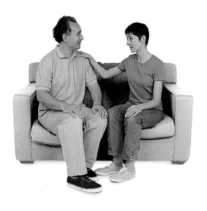

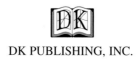

DK PUBLISHING, INC.

A DK PUBLISHING BOOK

Managing Editor	Jemima Dunne
Managing Art Editors	Philip Gilderdale and Lynne Brown
Project Editor	Dawn Bates
Editors	Caroline Fraser Ker, Nasim Mawji
US Editor	Jill Hamilton
Senior Art Editor	Karen Ward
Art Editor	Keith Davis
Designers	Sue Callister, Maria Wheatley
Production	Martin Croshaw
Photography	Andy Crawford

First American Edition, 1998
2 4 6 8 10 9 7 5 3 1
Published in the United States by DK Publishing, Inc.
95 Madison Avenue, New York, NY 10016
Visit us on the World Wide Web at http://www.dk.com

Library of Congress Cataloging-in-Publication Data

Caregiver's handbook / Visiting Nurse Associations. -- 1st American ed.
p. cm.
Includes index
ISBN 0-7894-1969-6
1. Home care services--United States--Handbooks, manuals, etc.
I. Visiting Nurse Associations of America
RA645.35.C37 1998
362.1'4--dc21   97-35911
                                                            CIP

Reproduced by Flying Colours SRL, Italy
Printed in Hong Kong by WKT

Publisher's note
The risks associated with lifting and handling tasks covered in this book are complex and each
situation must be judged on its own merits. Do not follow the instructions given in this book
without proper assessment of the individual circumstances.

FOREWORD

MANY OF US, AT SOME TIME IN OUR LIVES, will be in the position of caring for someone else. For some people, however, this caregiving role becomes a larger part of their lives, taking up more of their time because someone close has become sick or disabled. The decision to take on the many responsibilities of caregiving is an individual one, which involves both the needs of the person being cared for and the availability of the caregiver, as well as the relationship between the two people. This caregiving role is found throughout the world, transcending political, geographic, and social boundaries.

It is only in recent years that the role of caregivers has been recognized. Many services exist to help caregivers fulfill their role, but it is often difficult to take full advantage of all that is available. The need for information has led to CAREGIVER'S HANDBOOK, which gives advice on basic caregiving skills, plus an introduction to some of the financial and legal issues involved and suggestions on where to go to find further help.

The book has been written by a group of volunteers and paid staff from volunteer aid societies, all experienced caregivers themselves, with guidance from the Visiting Nurse Associations of America. It is written not only for caregivers but also for the volunteers who help and assist them.

We all need support and advice when we find ourselves in a position of providing care. It is our sincere hope that this book will provide some of that help to the many unsung heroes who take time out of their own lives to be caregivers.

Visiting Nurse Associations of America

CONTENTS

INTRODUCTION

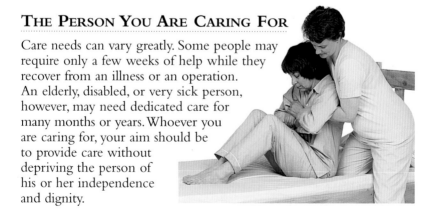

More and more people are being cared for at home, both because hospitals discharge patients more quickly and people live longer. There are millions of caregivers in the US who look after a sick, disabled, or elderly person at home. This book is the first illustrated guide to address their needs.

BEING A CAREGIVER

People become caregivers for different reasons. You may have chosen to look after a relative at home because he or she has come to depend on you and you do not want him or her to live in a nursing home or hospital. Alternatively, you may be a volunteer caregiver who has chosen to give your own time to provide help in the community. Whatever your situation, this book gives you the information you need so that you can provide the best and most rewarding care.

This book outlines and complements the support that you can obtain from federal and state health and social service agencies. We strongly suggest that you make the most of this help and any financial benefits because access to the right information and resources can help you to improve your quality of life and that of the person you are caring for.

THE PERSON YOU ARE CARING FOR

Care needs can vary greatly. Some people may require only a few weeks of help while they recover from an illness or an operation. An elderly, disabled, or very sick person, however, may need dedicated care for many months or years. Whoever you are caring for, your aim should be to provide care without depriving the person of his or her independence and dignity.

How This Book Can Help You

This definitive guide to home caregiving offers practical advice, emotional support, and essential information to help you provide the best quality of care possible.

Practical advice Step-by-step photographs show you the best ways to carry out day-to-day tasks, such as giving a bedbath or moving someone safely, with advice on equipment that can help you. Also shown are a wide range of aids, such as adapted kitchen utensils, that allow and encourage a physically impaired person to become more independent.

Emotional support The emotional difficulties that both you and your relative may face are addressed and solutions are offered. Case studies are used to highlight – and help you overcome – some of these difficulties. The expert, reassuring advice will guide you through distressing or uncomfortable situations.

Essential information There is a comprehensive guide to the resources available to you and your relative, from support groups to financial benefits.

A Guide to the Terms Used	
Gender: throughout the book, we refer to the person being cared for as "he" or "she" alternately from chapter to chapter, except in text that relates directly to an image.	
Relative	The person being cared for. This term is used because most people are related to the person they are caring for. The information in this book, however, is equally relevant if you are caring for a friend or a neighbor.
Home caregiver	Any person caring for a relative, friend, or neighbor in the home environment.
Volunteer caregiver	Anyone working as a caregiver for a volunteer organization. The yellow-tinted pages in the book specifically address the needs of the volunteer caregiver.
Care/ healthcare professional	A member of the professional care team. The chart on pages 10–11 gives details of the professionals and the services that they provide.

CARE PROFESSIONALS

THE CHART BELOW OUTLINES THE PROFESSIONALS with whom you may come into contact while you are caring for your relative. The actual job titles may vary from region to region; the possible alternatives are given in parentheses. A clinically trained care professional, such as an internist, nurse practitioner, or occupational therapist, is known as a "healthcare professional."

CARE PROFESSIONALS AND WHAT THEY DO

CARE PROFESSIONAL	LOCATION	SERVICES PROVIDED
Social worker (may also be called case worker)	Health center/ hospital/home health agency	Assesses the needs of the caregiver and the person being cared for. Produces a care plan and guidance on how to obtain services. Coordinates and monitors the care that is provided.
Internist	Health center/ physician's office	A physician who provides general medical advice and treatment, and can refer patients to a specialist, if necessary.
Geriatrician	Health center/ physician's office	A physician with special training in the diagnosis, treatment, and prevention of disorders in older people.
Surgeon	Hospital	A physician who treats disorders by operating. Many surgeons specialize on one part of the body.
Nurse practitioner	Health center/ physician's office	Has advanced education and training. Provides general nursing care and may in some regions, diagnose minor complaints and prescribe medicine.
Registered nurse	Health center/ physician's office/ home health agency	Supports the work of the physician, including doing a health assessment, and advising on diet and lifestyle. Carries out clinical procedures, such as wound dressings and injections.
Community psychiatric nurse/ Community mental health nurse	Health center or hospital psychiatric unit	Provides support and counseling for those with psychiatric problems; administers medication and monitors overall care and treatment given.

CARE PROFESSIONALS AND WHAT THEY DO

CARE PROFESSIONAL	LOCATION	SERVICES PROVIDED
Psychiatric social worker	Social Services or hospital psychiatric unit	Assesses social needs and provides help with practical problems, such as helping a person to fill in an application form for benefits.
Occupational therapist	Social Services	Assesses a person's individual requirements and advises on adapting the home, equipment, and activities to enable him or her to relearn skills and be self-sufficient.
Physical therapist	Social Services	Treats those with bone and joint problems. Advises on mobility and exercise.
Speech-language pathologist	Health center/hospital	Treats those with speech and language problems, including stroke victims.
Continence adviser	Health center/hospital	Provides advice and support, including recommending aids, for those with continence problems.
Stoma care nurse	Health center/hospital	Provides advice – on skin care and diet, for example – and support for a person who has a stoma.
Registered dietician	Health center/hospital/physician's office	Advises on nutrition and healthy diets; tailors special diets to suit specific medical conditions, such as diabetes.
Oncological care nurse	Hospital/hospice	Advises on pain and symptom control for cancer patients. Offers care, support, and counseling for patients and caregivers. Organizes short-term care to enable the caregiver to take a break.
Diabetic liaison nurse	Hospital or physician's office	Advises on the effective control of diabetes, as well as overall health matters.
Podiatrist	Hospital/health center	Offers specialist treatment and therapy for foot problems.
Ambulance personnel	Hospital/Fire department	Provide emergency treatment and transportation to the hospital.

VOLUNTEER ORGANIZATIONS

VOLUNTEER ORGANIZATIONS play an essential part in assisting and complementing the work of caregivers and health and social services. They provide care at all levels, ranging from helping those recently discharged from the hospital, to looking after sick, disabled, and elderly people. Each community is unique in the availability of service organizations and support groups. These can be found either in your local phone directory or by calling your state Area Agency on Aging (for a complete state-by-state list, *see pages 176–77*). You can also obtain information from a variety of specialist organizations, for example, the American Red Cross, American Diabetes Association, Alzheimer's Association, American Heart Association, or American Cancer Society (*see pages 174–75*).

VISITING NURSE ASSOCIATIONS OF AMERICA

The Visiting Nurse Associations of America (VNAA) is a national nonprofit membership organization that represents more than 200 community-based home and community health care providers. Each of the Visiting Nurse Associations is governed by a volunteer Board of Directors.

The home care provided by Visiting Nurse Associations includes highly skilled and lifesaving services as well as assistance with daily routines such as bathing, dressing, and eating. Care is provided, regardless of ability to pay, by individual nurses or by multidisciplinary teams that may include registered nurses; home health aides; social workers; physical, occupational, and speech-language therapists; and volunteers. Visiting Nurse Associations offer a variety of healthcare services including case management, infusion therapy, chemotherapy, enterostomal therapy, chronic care, homemaker and chore services, mental health and psychiatric care, HIV/AIDS education and treatment, social services, nutritional counseling, and hospice and respite care.

CHAPTER 1

BEING A CAREGIVER

The decision to provide care at home for
a sick, disabled, or elderly relative is not one to be taken lightly.
Although caring for someone can be very rewarding, it can also
affect your home and family life, your work, and your
free time. If your relative has gradually come to depend on you,
you may have become a caregiver without realizing it.
It is just as important, in this situation, to decide whether
it is the best option for you. This chapter outlines all aspects of
being a caregiver, so that you can weigh the advantages and
disadvantages of looking after your relative at
home and make an informed decision about becoming a caregiver
or continuing to be one. It may also help you accept that caring at
home may not necessarily be the best option for you and your
relative. If you do reach this decision, your physician should be
able to advise you on alternative caregiving arrangements.

LOOKING AFTER YOURSELF

To fulfill your role as a caregiver, you need to
maintain your own physical and emotional health. In order to
manage this, you need to ask for help and take time off whenever
possible. This section shows you how to take advantage of the help
that may be available from friends, family, social services, and
volunteer organizations. Asking for help – and thereby sacrificing
less of your own time – can enhance your relationship with
the person you are caring for.

BECOMING A CAREGIVER

Y OUR ROLE AS A CAREGIVER, and the length of time it lasts, can vary. If your relative's decline is gradual (as with Alzheimer's disease), you may be prepared to become a caregiver but if his decline is sudden (due to a stroke, for example), you may not be ready either physically or emotionally. Whatever the level of care, make sure it is the right choice for both of you.

CASE STUDY

NAME: GRACE
AGE: 67

G race had been married to Stanley for 45 years. Stanley's health gradually declined and he came to depend more and more on his wife. He had minor accidents: a fall left him with a broken arm and he forgot food cooking on the stove, which nearly caused a fire.

Grace did not realize that she had become his caregiver until she became afraid to leave him alone in the house. Although she wanted to continue to look after him herself, she realized it would be beneficial to both of them if she asked for some help.

Her first step was to look to friends and relatives for help with household chores. Later, a care worker visited and, after a discussion with Grace, arranged for help, which alleviated much of the pressure.

THE LEVEL OF CARE

Your relative may be self-sufficient in many ways but unable to cope with more strenuous chores such as cleaning or shopping; this could mean that he needs your help for only a few hours each week. In more extreme situations, however, you may be looking after someone who requires help with basic needs, such as bathing and feeding; in these circumstances, you would be required to provide constant care.

SHORT-TERM CARE

A person recovering from an operation or a major illness will require a high level of care initially. A care plan outlining your relative's needs should be prepared (*see page 33*); if there is any job you think you cannot handle, you should tell the hospital or your relative's physician. At first, you may be required to help with day-to-day tasks such as cooking or, if your relative has mobility problems, to help him move from room to room. As he recovers, however, your responsibilities should decrease. Someone who has had a heart attack and is convalescing at home, for example, may require intensive support and care initially but will gradually regain his strength.

LONG-TERM CARE

If your relative's physical or mental abilities are permanently impaired, you should seriously consider the practicalities of caring for him at home. In most situations quite extensive care needs will have to be considered. Full-time care may be required and may involve adaptations being made to your home – for example, a stairlift may have to be installed, or a downstairs room may have to be converted into a bedroom (*see* Adapting the Home, *pages 43–52*).

IS HOME CARE A PRACTICAL OPTION?

Caring for a relative can be a big responsibility that may affect nearly every aspect of your life. If you have been working outside the home, you may be able to obtain medical leave to take care of your relative (*see right*); otherwise, some form of medical reimbursement may be available. Remember, home care is not the only option available to you: if you have doubts, there are other alternatives. Before you decide whether to become a caregiver, consider the questions below.

YOU AND YOUR RELATIVE

◆ Will your relative require long- or short-term care?
◆ Will he need constant supervision?
◆ How does he feel about you being his caregiver?
◆ Are you the best person to be his caregiver?
◆ How much help can you get from friends, family, volunteer agencies, and social services?
◆ What other options are available if you don't become the caregiver?

YOUR PARTNER AND CHILDREN

◆ How will others in your household be affected?
◆ Can you fulfill your responsibilities to your relative, as well as to your partner and your children?
◆ Have you discussed the situation and made the decision as a family?

YOUR HOME

◆ Will you need to adapt your home?
◆ If so, will the changes be expensive? Are you eligible for aid (*see page 45*)?

WORK AND FINANCES

◆ Is it possible to get short-term medical leave?
◆ Are you prepared to give up your job, if necessary?
◆ Will either of you receive benefits (*see pages 164–68*)?

REASSESSING YOUR DECISION

Your relative's condition may improve or decline over time, affecting his level of dependence on you. Symptoms and circumstances change continually, so you should not feel obligated to stand by your original decision – you can reconsider the above factors at later stages.

DETERMINING YOUR CAREGIVING NEEDS

If you are employed outside the home, you are entitled as a caregiver to up to 12 weeks of unpaid, job-protected leave under the Family and Medical Leave Act of 1993. Medical leave is available to take care of a child, spouse, or parent who has a serious health condition that involves inpatient care in the hospital, a hospice, or a residential health care facility, or continuing treatment by the health care provider.

How your needs are assessed A social worker will talk to you about how you are coping, and will ask you what help is needed. Once your requirements have been determined, a care package will be designed that reflects both your needs and your relative's.

What may be provided To give you time off, a volunteer caregiver or sitter may be suggested. Your relative may be need specialized medical help (*see pages 10–11*). Advice may also be offered on any necessary changes to your home and on acquiring any appropriate specialized equipment.

BENEFITS OF HOME CARE

ALTHOUGH BEING A CAREGIVER is never easy – and there may be times when you will despair – it can be a most rewarding and satisfying experience. There will be demands and challenges to meet, and you may find that you are forced to draw on previously hidden reserves of strength. Caregiving can also be a fulfilling experience since your relative benefits from the care you provide.

CASE STUDY

NAME: FRANK
AGE: 42

Frank gave up his full-time job to look after his wife, Marjorie, when she became ill with cancer. He and Marjorie had often joked about his culinary skills, which did not stretch beyond boiling an egg. Now, suddenly, he found himself in the position of having to learn how to do everything – look after the children and get them to school on time, cook, do the housework and the shopping – and all on an income that was considerably reduced.

Frank discovered that caring for Marjorie, the children, and the home was a full-time job in itself. He also started to understand more about life at home. The experience of caring for his wife and sharing many of the routine tasks brought the whole family closer together.

BENEFITS FOR YOU

Your role as a caregiver is ultimately one of giving, but do not forget that there are also benefits for you.
Emotional strength Your relative is likely to rely on you for comfort and support when he is in low spirits and in need of reassurance. You may find that the emotional support you provide strengthens your relationship, bringing you closer together.
Pride You should take pride and satisfaction in the fact that your relative is receiving the best care that you can provide.
Organizational skills Looking after another person requires you to prioritize and organize your time efficiently; these skills can stand you in good stead throughout your life.

BENEFITS FOR YOUR RELATIVE

You are uniquely placed to provide your relative with a quality of life that may not be possible elsewhere.
Independence You can plan your time and structure a typical day together, which gives your relative a level of control and freedom that he might not receive in a more ordered environment, such as a residential home.
Personal care The smallest things, from knowing the type of soap your relative prefers to preparing his favorite meal, can make an immense difference to his quality of life. Maintaining some semblance of normal home life can be very reassuring for him.
Comfort Being cared for at home allows your relative to be in familiar surroundings, close to the people and things he knows and loves. He may be reassured to know that you are nearby to lend emotional support whenever he needs it. He may also want to be close to a pet, such as a dog or cat.

HOW RELATIONSHIPS CHANGE

C ARING FOR SOMEONE can affect your relationship with that person and other people to whom you are close. When someone who was previously fit and healthy becomes dependent because of an illness or disability, power balances shift and roles within a relationship inevitably change. By the same token, some relationships are fortified by the intimacy and closeness that caregiving brings.

CARING FOR YOUR PARENT

Most of us look up to our parents and rely on them for love and support, even when we have families of our own. It can be very distressing when the person you have always relied upon becomes frail or sick, and you may feel that you should assume responsibility for looking after him. When a parent's health deteriorates, we are all reminded of our mortality. In such situations, role reversal is inevitable but not easy for anyone to accept. It may be difficult for a father to accept that he is no longer the protector and provider, and must look to you for care. You, on the other hand, may feel you are being pressured into a caregiving role, and you may feel guilty for wanting to avoid the responsibility. For many, however, caring for a parent offers an opportunity to repay them for their help over the years.

CARING FOR A CHILD

When a child becomes severely sick or is disabled, the possibility that he may have to forego normal development and therefore he may not have the same opportunities as other children can cause overwhelming grief. Your instinct will probably be to overprotect your child but, where possible, you should encourage him to do things for himself. Contacting a specialist organization (*see pages 175–76*) to learn about his illness or disability, and the limitations it will impose, may help you cope. For example, with the right support, a child with Down's syndrome may develop skills that will enable him to lead a full life. The specialist organization may also be able to put you in touch with other parents caring for children who have the same illness or disability.

CASE STUDY
NAME: JOHN
AGE: 27

J **ohn** discovered that he was HIV-positive and desperately wanted to tell his parents, but he dreaded their reaction – his father's in particular. His father had never been able to accept the fact that his son was homosexual and this had been the source of much anger and hostility between them.

When John developed AIDS, his mother insisted that he move home so that she could care for him. This forced them to accept what was happening and to reassess their relationship.

John's return home saw the beginning of a new understanding between him and his parents as they all began to realize that there was no point in punishing one another with recriminations, but that they had to try to accept one another as they were.

THE EFFECTS ON YOUR FAMILY

If your relative comes to live with you, try to involve your partner and your children in his care. This will ease some of the strain on you and will help your relative to feel that he is part of the household. Your family may be affected in different ways.

Children They may feel neglected, even jealous, especially if you have to devote more of your time to your relative and less to them. Try to make time for them and, if they want to, involve them in helping to care for your relative.

Partner Make time for your partner; he too may feel neglected. Try not to take out your frustrations on him, and be as honest and open as possible with each other: hiding your feelings will put an unnecessary strain on your relationship.

Your sex life may be affected: the physical and emotional exhaustion of being a caregiver can in itself be enough to kill sexual desire. Discuss this with your partner and reassure him that your feelings have not changed.

CARING FOR YOUR PARTNER

Most couples entertain a romantic dream of growing old together. Whether sudden or gradual, the transition of one partner into being a caregiver brings inevitable change within a relationship: one partner needs to provide more care and support while the other becomes increasingly dependent. It may be a difficult time and you may both have to learn to cope with feelings of sadness: you because the person you love is ill; your partner because he has to adjust to this new, unexpected role of being a dependent.

COPING WITH TASKS

When an illness is physically debilitating, you may have to minister to your partner on quite an intimate level. This may bring you closer together, but you may also find it awkward and embarrassing and want to consider enlisting outside help.

UNDERSTANDING YOUR FEELINGS

If your partner has an illness that affects him mentally, such as Alzheimer's disease, there may be times when you feel that you have lost sight of the person you fell in love with, and become frustrated and angry because you can no longer communicate as you used to. There may even be times when you feel hurt, insulted, or angry because your partner becomes confused and does not recognize you. These are natural feelings; if you become exasperated, speak to someone who can understand.

ADAPTING TO A CHANGED SEXUAL RELATIONSHIP

It may be that your partner's illness has changed him physically and that this has affected your sexual relationship. If so, it is important that you share your feelings openly. He may feel ashamed or awkward, and, if he senses that you are becoming distant, it will only reinforce his feelings of isolation. Sex is an important part of a relationship, but people are often shy about discussing it, worrying in silence rather than seeking advice. Sexual desire does ebb, and at times your levels of desire may not be compatible. If you and your partner cannot talk openly, ask your physician to recommend someone who can help.

LOOKING AFTER YOURSELF

As a CAREGIVER, you have responsibilities to yourself as well as to the person for whom you are caring. Looking after your physical health and being conscientious about your own diet, exercise, and sleep will keep you strong and help you maintain your emotional resilience. If your own health begins to suffer, you will not be able to help either your relative or yourself.

DIET

If you are busy and your relative has little appetite, you may be tempted to skip regular meals and exist on snacks. Consider the suggestions below as ways of finding time to enjoy a meal:

◆ Invite a friend or relative over to share a meal. This will provide a break, as well as some company; it may also inspire you to prepare a meal.

◆ When inviting a friend, or even a group of friends, suggest that everyone contribute a dish to the meal.

EXERCISE

Even though you are physically active as a caregiver, you should try to make time for regular exercise away from home. This will make you feel more energetic, and provide a break from your daily activities. Consider the following exercise options.

Exercise classes A class can provide a regular break in your routine; it may also be refreshing to meet people not involved in caregiving. Can you set aside a block of time each week and be sure that you can keep to it? Could you arrange for a friend to sit with your relative for a couple of hours while you attend a yoga class? Could you go to an exercise class while your relative is at a day center?

Swimming and walking Timewise, these activities are much more flexible and demand a lower level of commitment than classes. Although more solitary, it may suit you better just to switch off and swim a few lengths of the pool or go for a walk in the park.

Exercising together Is there any way your relative could accompany you to the sports center? Some local pools run swimming classes for disabled people; this may be a way for you to exercise at the same time.

DO'S & DON'TS

Looking after yourself is an essential part of caring for someone else.

☑ **Do** get enough sleep (*see page 20*).

☑ **Do** discuss plans for dieting (to lose weight) with your physician. As a caregiver, your energy requirements may differ from someone else of your age and build.

☑ **Do** drink plenty of fluids, especially fruit juices.

☑ **Do** eat plenty of fresh fruit and vegetables.

☑ **Do** moderate your alcohol and cigarette consumption.

☒ **Don't** use alcohol or cigarettes as a crutch in stressful moments.

☒ **Don't** snack on cakes and cookies to maintain energy levels.

☒ **Don't** forego proper, regular meals. This is easy to do, but is not good for you in the long term.

UNDERSTANDING EMOTIONS

C AREGIVING CAN BE EMOTIONALLY DRAINING, and you may not always be able to maintain a positive outlook. There may be times when you are confused by your feelings, or even ashamed, but the worst thing you can do is to bottle them up. The first step to understanding your feelings is to identify them; it is only then that you can find ways of working them out.

ALLEVIATING TIREDNESS

There is nothing more likely than tiredness and exhaustion to fray your temper and make you irritable. Think about ways in which you can alleviate tiredness.

Planning your day
Draw up a list of your typical daily tasks, then prioritize them. Are they all absolutely necessary? Could you delegate some of them to family or friends? For example, could someone else do the ironing while you have a short rest?

Getting adequate rest
If your relative sleeps in the afternoon, you should try to nap then too. If you have trouble getting to sleep at night, the following tips may help:
♦ try to keep a regular bedtime routine;

♦ keep the bedroom at a comfortable temperature;

♦ avoid stimulants such as caffeine before bedtime;

♦ don't go to bed hungry.

IDENTIFYING STRESS

It is difficult to avoid becoming stressed; you may often feel that there are not enough hours in the day and that there is no end in sight to the jobs you have to tackle. You may become irritable and moody and feel constantly tired. You may find that on some days even the simplest of tasks, such as washing up, is just too much to handle. By identifying the signs of stress early on and dealing with them, you can limit their destructive effects.

RECOGNIZING AND OVERCOMING STRESS
When you recognize the first signs of stress, try the following stress-reducing tips:
♦ Breathe in deeply and slowly through your nose and out through your mouth. Repeat ten times.
♦ When you are offered time off, use it to spoil yourself. Try not to think about household tasks you could be doing. Get out of the house: visit a favorite place, see a movie, have your hair done, or see friends.
♦ If you can't get out, have a long, relaxing bath with essential oils or bath salts. Read a magazine or listen to your favorite music.
♦ Make sure that you go to bed at a reasonable hour, if possible, and that you get enough sleep (*see left*).
♦ Try to get some exercise during the day. If you can't get out of the house, is there an exercise program on television or video that you can do? Gentle exercise, such as stretching, may be good for both you and your relative, and may be something you can do together; it may even be a source of laughter.
♦ Talk to someone about how you are feeling and, if it helps, have a good cry. A friend, your physician, a specialist organization, or a relevant support group (*see pages 175–76*) may be able to listen and help.

UNDERSTANDING ANGER AND GUILT

It is only human to feel angry when something happens that hurts you or upsets your plans. This is a natural and healthy response, especially when someone you love falls ill or becomes disabled. Anger is a complex emotion, and it is often suppressed because we feel guilty about expressing it. If you can get to the root of your anger, you will have gone part of the way toward dealing with it, as well as with the accompanying guilt. There are certainly times when anger needs to be controlled, but it should never be ignored. Here are some of the common reasons why you, as a caregiver, may experience anger and guilt:

♦ someone you love is suffering;
♦ the illness or disability has upset all your future plans together, and you feel guilty about feeling angry;
♦ you are angry at your relative for being sick and, even though you know this is irrational, it does not stop you from feeling this way;
♦ you feel that the situation is unjust, that neither you nor your relative deserves what is happening;
♦ it may be an expression of the frustration you feel as a caregiver – you may feel that you cannot cope.

CASE STUDY

NAME: HARRY AGE: 72

Harry, who cared for his wife Margaret – who was suffering from Parkinson's disease – began to feel increasingly angry and isolated. The family physician suggested that he contact a caregivers' support group so that he could talk to others in similar situations.

Harry confessed to a caregiver who visited him that he sometimes felt angry because Margaret could no longer do the things she had once been able to, and sometimes did not even recognize him. He felt angry because his wife was slow and uncommunicative, then he felt guilty because he knew she could not help it. The visiting caregiver told him that she, too, had felt anger and the grief that came with seeing someone you love deteriorate.

Harry now relies on the group for support; he knows that there are other caregivers he can talk to who will understand his frustration about doing everything he can for Margaret, but never feeling that it is quite enough.

DO'S AND DON'TS

Anger can get out of control and lead to irrational judgments and decisions, even violence.

✓ **Do** discuss your problems with the care professional or physician; either may refer you to someone who can help.

✓ **Do** seek the help of a specialist organization (*see pages 175–76*) that pertains to your relative's illness; they will be able to empathize with your situation and offer both you and your relative advice and support.

✓ **Do** get away from your relative for a few minutes if you feel yourself getting tense. First, make sure he can be safely left on his own.

✓ **Do** try to understand that your relative may feel angry and frustrated at times. He may also feel guilty about having to rely on you so much.

✗ **Don't** cut yourself off from friends because you are angry at them for not sharing your suffering. You will only isolate yourself further and become embittered.

✗ **Don't** be ashamed of your anger. Talk about your feelings before they become overwhelming.

SEEKING COUNSELING

Caregivers often face problems that seem insurmountable.

Can counseling help?
Counseling is one way of helping people adjust and come to terms with their difficulties; it is also good for exploring practical ways to solve problems. Counseling is not a "cure" for people with psychiatric or physical illnesses and it is not psychotherapy, which is a treatment for people with specific mental health problems.

Choosing a counselor
The availability of counseling varies widely across the country, and choosing a counselor can be difficult. Some private counselors advertise their services; others are associated with volunteer organizations such as the American Red Cross. The American Counseling Association (*see page 174*) can supply a list of counselors in your area. Increasingly, counselors are attached to medical offices to facilitate insurance coverage. Your physician should also be able to assess your needs and refer you to a psychiatrist or psychologist if needed.

COPING WITH LONELINESS AND ISOLATION

It is easy to become isolated as a caregiver. You may find that you are too busy to keep up with friends and relatives. If people visit less frequently, it may be because they see that you are busy, and worry that they may be in the way. Sometimes people stop visiting because they are embarrassed about your relative's illness. The following positive steps may help:
◆ Make time to contact people and reassure them that you still need their friendship and support.
◆ Try to be open and honest about your feelings and your needs – don't shut people out or try to pretend that you can cope on your own. To feel happy in your caregiving role you need to feel supported and loved.
◆ Be open about your relative's illness and what it means in terms of daily care.
◆ Offer reassurance to people if they are frightened or upset by the signs of the illness – remember that they are not as familiar as you are with the situation.
◆ Enlist the help of friends and relatives, and involve them in the care if you can. People are often happier if they know they are making a positive contribution.

RECOGNIZING DEPRESSION

There may well be times when everything gets on top of you, when you don't know where you will find the resolve to go on. Normally these feelings will pass if you talk to a friend, get a good night's sleep, or take a break. Sometimes, however, they persist and develop into depression, which can be destructive. Some of the more common symptoms of depression you should watch out for are:
◆ tearfulness
◆ irritability
◆ tiredness
◆ feelings of inadequacy
◆ lack of concentration
◆ fitful sleep, or too much sleep
◆ eating all the time, or complete loss of appetite
If you are experiencing any of these symptoms and you feel that you can't discuss your feelings with a friend, you might want to consider seeking impartial advice from a counselor or physician (*see left*).

FINDING TIME FOR YOURSELF

LOOKING AFTER SOMEONE FULL TIME is a demanding job. At times you will need a break, not only from daily chores, but also from your relative, for a few hours, a day, a week, or longer. To do this you will need respite care. Respite care ranges from someone sitting with your relative for an afternoon or your relative going into a residential home for a short stay.

MAKING TIME FOR YOURSELF

You may feel guilty about wanting to take a break because you think it implies that you do not care about your relative. However, there are many reasons why it is *essential* to take time away from caregiving.
To reduce stress levels Being stressed will mean that you are more prone to illness, irritability, and depression. Caregivers often struggle on unaided, denying themselves any relief until their own health suffers. Time off can help put things in perspective.
To improve your caregiving relationship To keep a relationship alive and interesting, you need to talk to other people and have other experiences. Your relationship with your relative is no different: time apart will almost certainly give both of you new perspectives and different things to talk about.
For your independence Your relative is necessarily dependent on you, the caregiver, but remember that you also need care, not least in the form of emotional support. Spend time keeping up with friends and family and maintaining your own social life. Try to find time for a hobby, if you have one. Retaining some degree of independence will mean that you are less likely to become isolated and feel overwhelmed.

ARRANGING RESPITE CARE

You can arrange a short break yourself (for example, by asking a friend to care for your relative for the afternoon), but help can also be provided by social services, your local community medical center, and volunteer associations. The care provided, and who provides it, will depend on the severity of your relative's condition. You might also consider a care attendant, who provides care in the home. For respite care options, see the chart on pages 24–25.

RESIDENTIAL RESPITE CARE

If you are thinking of taking a break for a week or more, one option is for your relative to go to stay in a residential care home. Consider the following when you are choosing a temporary care home:

◆ Does it have a current state license?

◆ Are the staff experienced in dealing with your relative's particular needs?

◆ Does your relative like the place?

◆ Is it well kept and clean?

◆ How is the food?

◆ Are the staff friendly?

◆ Are any temporary residents fully integrated into the life of the home? Are they included in outings?

◆ Are there others having a temporary break?

◆ Is the nursing home comfortably furnished and tastefully decorated?

RESPITE CARE

THE BEST TYPE OF RESPITE CARE for your relative will depend on his particular requirements, the length of time you will be away, and the cost involved. Cost and availability will vary according to the area in which you live. If you require only a short break, it may be worth asking family and friends for help in caring for your relative.

TYPE OF CARE	LENGTH OF BREAK	SERVICES PROVIDED
Day center	A day or more a week, as required.	This will vary from center to center, but may include occupational therapy such as art, amateur dramatics, fitness classes, and craft work. Services such as hairdressing may also be available.
Hospital	As required.	Complete medical and nursing care, including rehabilitation. Some hospitals offer clergy and/or spiritual support.
Hospice/Inpatient	According to requirements, it could be from days to weeks.	Pain and symptom relief, clergy and/or spiritual support, counseling service, and alternative therapies (e.g., massage). Home-sitting service may be available.
Nursing home/ residential care home	1–2 weeks.	This will vary from home to home, but may include occupational therapy such as art, amateur dramatics, fitness classes, and craft work. Services such as podiatry may also be available.
Sitting service	Day or night, as arranged.	Day or night nursing, general care and supervision.
Volunteer help	A few hours/daily.	Outings or home help.
Private nurse	Depends on means and requirements.	Any nursing care appropriate to your relative's requirements, from changing dressings and giving injections to giving a bath.
Assisted living	Depends on means and requirements.	For those who can live on their own but need some supervision, as well as help with meals, laundry, and other personal and housekeeping chores.

How Can Family and Friends Help?

Some people will be anxious to help but may be unsure as to exactly how. Here are some suggestions:

◆ Could someone sit with your relative for a few hours to give you a chance to rest or go out?

◆ Could a family member come and stay occasionally, or could your relative go and stay with him or her?

◆ Could someone help with the ironing, vacuuming, laundry, or washing?

◆ Could anyone help with small tasks such as shopping or picking up a prescription?

Level of Care	Where to Find Out What is Available
From attendant to registered nurse, but it depends on staffing levels and whether or not people with certain conditions are catered for.	Social services, volunteer organizations, library, local press, and physician's office, local hospital, or medical center. Local area agency on aging (*see pages 174, 176–77*).
Physicians and registered nurses. Social worker. Specialist help, such as physical therapy.	Referral from your relative's physician.
Full care with specialist doctors, registered nurses, and complementary medicine specialists.	Social services, referral from your relative's physician, community nursing, local paper, library. Admittance normally limited to those with cancer or those who are terminally ill.
Residential care home: usually care assistants with additional medical cover by physicians and nurse practitioners. Nursing home: the above and registered nurses.	Social services, referral from your relative's physician, local paper, library, support groups, volunteer organizations. Social services in some areas may help with fees.
Volunteers or registered nurses.	Social services, volunteer organizations, support groups, hospices, community nursing services.
May not be specialized. Depends on your relative's requirements.	Neighbor, friends, family, support groups, volunteer organizations.
Registered nurse.	Nursing agency, physician. Cost may be a limitation because private nurses can be expensive.
Trained staff, including nurses and custodians, are available in most assisted living arrangements.	Local area agency on aging or long-term care ombudsman. The Department of Consumer Affairs or the Better Business Bureau can tell you whether any complaints have been filed.

GOING ON VACATION TOGETHER

C ARING FOR YOUR RELATIVE does not mean that you have to be permanently confined to the home. Respite vacations enable your relative to have a vacation – in the care of someone else – thereby also giving you a break. If you want to go on vacation together, contact one of the organizations that arranges vacations for those with special care needs.

FACILITIES CHECKLIST

Before booking a vacation, check that the facilities are suitable for your relative's needs:

◆ Are all areas – such as dining room, gardens, and elevators – accessible by wheelchair?

◆ Is the accommodation accessible to someone with limited mobility? Is your relative's room on the ground floor?

◆ Is there an elevator/ stairlift?

◆ Are there facilities for disabled people, such as handrails in the toilet and shower?

◆ Are there bed and bathtub hoists?

◆ Are the beds adjustable and electrically operated?

◆ Are there facilities for guide dogs?

◆ Are registered nurses, care assistants, or trained medical staff available?

◆ Are treatments, such as physical therapy or hydrotherapy, available?

CHOOSING A VACATION

Vacations that cater specifically for the needs of sick or disabled people are available: these provide different levels of care depending on individual needs.

PLANNING AHEAD

Make sure you discuss any special needs and the level of care required with the tour operator beforehand (*see left*). Most can offer useful information, such as the location of specially built vacation centers and whether or not there are caregivers on hand to assist with daily care, such as helping someone to eat.

CONTACTING SPECIALIST ORGANIZATIONS

In the US, contact the Society for the Advancement of Travel for the Handicapped (SATH) (*see page 174*), which provides information about low-cost vacations with accommodation and transportation facilities for sick or disabled people. The aim of the service is to give caregivers and their relatives the confidence to travel away from home. To ensure a current database of the level of care available, the Society works closely with vacation and tour operators. The International Association for Medical Assistance to Travelers (IMAT) has coordinated English-speaking doctors throughout the world to provide assistance to travelers requiring medical assistance while away from home.

GETTING THERE

A local volunteer organization may be able to assist with travel arrangements, such as transportation, or the travel company may be able to organize this. Most railroads offer help, and airlines are required to give "on and off" assistance, and help at airports, to people who have mobility problems.

SUPPORT GROUPS

PEOPLE WHO SHARE EXPERIENCES of a particular disease or disability often form groups so that they can offer support and understanding to each other, and share tips on how to cope. There are two types of support group: those formed to provide information about a particular condition, offering help to you and your relative, and those that are there to support the caregiver.

WHY JOIN A SUPPORT GROUP?

By joining a support group you can benefit from meeting new people in a similar situation to yourself and offer and receive help and advice.

To meet others in a similar situation The life of a caregiver can be a very isolated one: meeting and sharing your experiences with others in the same position can be life-affirming in itself.

To have a break It is understandable to want time away from your caregiving role. Support groups often find someone to stay with your relative, and may arrange your transportation to and from the meeting.

To obtain information If an illness is rare and experience in dealing with the symptoms is limited, support groups can provide an opportunity for caregivers and their relatives to meet and pool their knowledge. These groups often offer specialized training as well. Support groups can also keep you up-to-date regarding benefits and your rights as a caregiver.

For support Members are usually caregivers, ex-caregivers, or sufferers themselves, so they are well placed to understand your problems and offer practical advice and support. Because they are or have been in your position, they will be able to identify with your feelings and will reassure you that you are not alone.

FINDING THE RIGHT SUPPORT GROUP

Many support groups are formed specifically for people coping with or caring for someone with a particular disease or disability. There are also many more general groups; for example, the American Association for Retired Persons campaigns on issues such as benefits, recognition, and support for all caregivers. They have a main office and a network of local groups nationwide (*see page 174*).

FORMING A SUPPORT GROUP

If you cannot find a suitable group, consider starting one yourself: the National Association for Home Care provides a free information pack.

Get others interested Advertise locally for others with similar experiences. The nurse practitioner or physician may be able to help you start a group.

Arrange a meeting Fix a date, a time, and a suitable venue, for example, a physician's office or town hall.

Clarify your aims Is there a particular cause you wish to champion or do you just want to meet people in the same position as yourself?

Confidentiality Agree on confidentiality from the start. No one will feel relaxed if they worry that their experiences may be discussed outside the group.

ARE YOU COPING?

I T IS POSSIBLE THAT YOU AND YOUR RELATIVE may find that home care is not practical. While many adapt easily to the role of home caregiver, some, understandably, find it difficult to cope. Bear in mind, too, that circumstances may have changed and it may be time to look at alternatives for care. It is important, however, that both of you are happy with the final decision.

PINPOINTING PROBLEMS

It may help to draw up a rough schedule detailing your daily care duties. You can then use this information to get a perspective on a typical week and to pinpoint areas where you need help. An early morning routine might look something like this:

◆ 7am Get up; wash and have breakfast.

◆ 7:30 Get Anna up, give her breakfast.

◆ 8:30 Help Anna into the bathtub and help her bathe.

◆ 9:15 Dress Anna.

◆ 9:30 Dress myself, then do some housework.

Do you need help in the mornings? Has it become too much of a physical strain to move your relative, for example? Seek advice from a care professional who may be able to help you assess the situation and find alternative ways of meeting your care needs.

ASSESSING YOUR SITUATION

To find out if home care is still a practical option for you, examine your day-to-day routine and consider how you are feeling physically and emotionally.

Organization Is there a routine to your day? Are you managing your time as efficiently as possible?

Priorities Are you wasting time and energy on unnecessary tasks and problems that will only increase your stress levels?

Support Are you getting all the help you can? Have you considered all your options: friends, relatives, volunteer organizations, and social services?

Financial entitlements Are you claiming the benefits to which you are entitled (*see pages 164–68*)?

Physical health Are you eating and sleeping properly? Are you able to exercise on a fairly regular basis?

Emotional health Are you able to maintain a rational outlook? Do you feel on top of things at most times? If not, do you have a friend or a counselor with whom you can share your feelings?

Breaks Are you getting enough time for yourself? Are you taking regular weekly breaks or vacations?

Independence Can you get out to see friends? Do you still have a social life?

Commitments Can you keep commitments to others in your family and to yourself?

A PERSPECTIVE ON YOUR DECISION

If at any stage you decide that you can no longer care for your relative at home, do not feel guilty or think that you have failed. It will probably be in the best interests for both of you if he is provided with alternative care, especially if he needs more specialized help and supervision than you are able to provide.

CHAPTER 2

BEING A VOLUNTEER

A volunteer may be required to look after a
person if there is no friend or relative to act as a caregiver.
A volunteer may also be required to help a home caregiver; either
to allow him to take time off or to help him with strenuous
tasks that he cannot do alone, such as helping his
relative get out of bed or into the bathtub.
The social services increasingly rely on volunteer
organizations, and the volunteer caregivers who work for them, to
provide both short- and long-term support.

THE ROLE OF THE VOLUNTEER

As a volunteer, you may be supervised
and supported by a care professional, such as a registered nurse,
who is responsible for determining and reviewing the
needs of the person and who will advise you on the
level of care that is required. Integral to your role is the ability to
get along with people – the person being cared for;
the home caregiver, if there is one; and
the professionals with whom you may work.
In order to provide the best service, you should feel fulfilled in
your role and be able to address problems and ask for help when
necessary. Being a volunteer can be hard work and is sometimes
very challenging, but ultimately it can be a highly
rewarding and satisfying experience.

BECOMING A VOLUNTEER

PEOPLE OF ALL AGES can volunteer to be caregivers – volunteer organizations welcome the help of anyone who is willing to give time to assist others. To make inquiries, telephone or write to your local library to request information about the type of volunteer caregiving taking place in your community, and for advice on how you can get involved.

CASE STUDY

NAME: PAUL
AGE: 18

Paul worked in a store. To widen his interests, Paul decided to volunteer in the community in his free time. He approached a local volunteer group and discovered that their activities ranged from organizing outings for young disabled people, to providing care in the home for sick, elderly, or disabled people.

After an initial discussion with the volunteer coordinator, Paul decided that he would like to help look after someone in the home. He received training in basic care skills, such as how to move and handle a person, and took a course in communication skills.

Being a caregiver made Paul more confident and better able to deal with people – skills that soon led to his promotion to supervisor at work.

WHAT DOES IT INVOLVE?

Becoming a volunteer caregiver may be a daunting prospect for many people. Below are some of the most common questions asked by potential volunteers.

WILL I BE INTERVIEWED?

You will probably be interviewed and asked for references, and you may be required to sign a form declaring that you do not have any health problems or a criminal record. You may also meet other volunteers in your area, who will explain the procedure for becoming a caregiver and what the work involves.

WHAT KIND OF WORK IS INVOLVED?

The type of work can vary from a couple of hours a day spent helping an elderly person with gardening, to sitting overnight with someone who is sick. You will never be expected to take on any task, or care for any person, if it makes you feel uncomfortable.

WHAT SKILLS DO I NEED?

You do not need any specialized skills to volunteer to be a caregiver. You will, however, be offered training ranging from how to communicate with a wide variety of people, to basic first-aid and caregiving skills. The skills gained as a volunteer will help you regardless of your economic background, and working in the community is respected by employers. The work may also be accredited to other training programs.

HOW MANY HOURS WILL I HAVE TO WORK?

The number of hours you agree to work is entirely up to you; you can arrange times to suit your lifestyle and other commitments. You can be flexible, but you must give notice if you cannot carry out your duties.

WORKING WITH PROFESSIONALS

YOU MAY BE REQUIRED to liaise with a number of professional people, such as registered nurses and social workers. These people are responsible for assessing the level of care needed by the person you are caring for, and making sure that it is carried out. When working with care professionals, you will be under their guidance, complementing rather than replacing their duties.

UNDERSTANDING YOUR ROLE

The care professional will delegate tasks to you or ask you to assist him. You may also be required to help a home caregiver to permit him to have some time off.

BEING RELIABLE

Reliability is a key element in your relations with professional care workers. If you cannot meet a commitment, you should always try to give plenty of notice so that alternative arrangements can be made. If you cancel at the last minute, or fail to turn up, you will be letting down the person being cared for and may be compromising the good name of the volunteer organization for which you work.

FOLLOWING A CARE PLAN

Social services may give you a care plan (*see page 33*) that has been devised following an assessment of the person requiring care. If you are given such a plan, you should always adhere to the recommendations made in it.

The type of care The requirements of the person being cared for and the kind of activities you will need to carry out.

The level of care The extent and frequency of the care you will give to that person.

The objectives of the care The specific aims the care plan is trying to achieve.

WHAT YOU CAN OFFER

You may see the person you are caring for more often than the care professional. If you notice improvements or a deterioration in the person's health, or recognize any deficiencies in the care plan, you should mention these and suggest possible changes.

CASE STUDY

NAME: EMMA
AGE: 32

Emma began caring for Mr. Thomas, who was confined to bed for most of the time because of a serious back injury. On her first visit, she referred to the care plan she had been given by the registered nurse. This stated that Mr. Thomas would require a bedbath, which Emma had been trained to do.

After she had cared for Mr. Thomas for a month, his condition improved. Based on her past experience, and after discussing it with him, Emma felt that he might now be fit enough to get into a bathtub by himself.

Emma knew it was not within the scope of her duties to change the care orders. However, she suggested it to the registered nurse, who reassessed Mr. Thomas's condition during her next visit and altered the care orders accordingly.

CARING FOR SOMEONE

EVEN THOUGH, AS A VOLUNTEER CAREGIVER, you are not a qualified professional, you should not think of yourself as an amateur. It is important that you act professionally so that the person you are caring for trusts you. Although you may become a close companion or a friend, you should still remember to behave responsibly and maintain confidentiality at all times.

HOME CAREGIVER

As a volunteer caregiver, you may be in close contact with a home caregiver. Since you must work well as a team, your relationship with that person is as critical as your relationship with the person you care for.

Practical support You can help with day-to-day tasks or provide nighttime care to give the home caregiver some time to himself. You can also make sure that he is aware of, and using, all the resources that are available to him. For example, he may welcome your help in obtaining advice and information about the financial benefits to which he may be entitled.

Emotional support The home caregiver may lead an isolated life, and may find the burden of caregiving very arduous. Just by being there to support and listen to him, you may help.

SATISFY THE NEEDS OF THE CARED FOR

The most important aspect of your volunteer role is to provide care without depriving the person of her independence and self-confidence.

Individuality The person being cared for has needs and preferences that should be respected. Try to understand why she may be acting in a certain way.

Independence Wherever possible, allow the person to make decisions and do things for herself, even if this means that a task takes longer. Always ask her opinion and respect her views.

Confidence If the person being cared for feels she is a burden to everyone, she will become lonely and insecure. Comfort and reassure her, and encourage her to focus on the skills and abilities that she has.

BE AWARE OF YOUR OWN LIMITATIONS

As a volunteer you will be giving much of your time to others, and may be dealing with stressful situations. If you are dissatisfied or unhappy, it will be difficult for you to provide the best care.

Having limited skills You may feel that you have not been fully trained or are not qualified to deal with some of the duties required of you, and that you are encroaching on the work of the care professional.

Feeling uncomfortable It may be that you don't get along with the person you are caring for, or feel ill at ease in the environment in which you are working.

Being unable to give enough You may feel that you are being asked to provide more care than you are able to offer. Try to recognize your own limitations and, if they affect the quality of the care you are providing, discuss them with your supervisor.

How a Care Plan Can Help You

When someone needs care, a plan is essential because it provides a clear list of the person's requirements. It can be used by other volunteer caregivers or care professionals who come into the home. The plan should be provided by a care professional, who may ask you to help devise it or, alternatively, to make recommendations. If, for any reason, it is not provided, request one from your supervisor or seek specific guidance about the type of care that the person requires. An example of a care plan is shown below.

CARE PLAN	NAME: *BETTY FRASER* AGE: *91*
ACTIVITY	ASSESSMENT
Mobility	*Mobile with the use of a cane. A wheelchair should be used for long distances.*
Bathing	*Can wash unaided; needs help to get into and out of the bathtub.*
Dressing	*Needs basic supervision.*
Eating	*Needs some help and encouragement. Prefers to eat with a spoon from a bowl, so cut up food or give soft foods if possible. Likes hot chocolate in the evening.*
Continence	*No problem.*
Sight	*Poor vision, even with eyeglasses.*
Hearing	*Adequate. Good with the use of an aid.*
Behavior	*Mildly confused at times. Should be informed about any visitors.*
Medication	*Twice daily for arthritis, with morning and evening meals.*
Communication	*Retains most information and indicates needs verbally.*
Finances	*Managed by her daughter.*
Social activities	*Enjoys joining arranged activities. Attends day center every other Wednesday.*
Hobbies	*Enjoys listening to the radio and having the newspaper read to her.*
Level of care	*Betty needs care twice daily from Monday to Friday (her daughter cares for her on weekends). She should be visited first thing in the morning and late in the afternoon. She receives Meals on Wheels at lunchtime, but her evening meal should be prepared for her.*
Objectives of care	*Betty is quite able, and should be encouraged to be independent. Regular attendance at a day center has been successful. Aim for attendance at least once a week by the end of the year.*

SIGNS OF ABUSE

Evidence suggests that abuse is more likely to be the result of poor preexisting relationships, or alcohol or mental health problems, rather than due to the strain of caregiving. Abuse does occur, however, and it could be either the caregiver or the cared for who is the abuser. If you suspect abuse of any kind, inform your supervisor, who will deal with it through the correct channels. Do not share your suspicions with anyone else.

Physical abuse Watch for signs such as bruising and negative body language (*see page 38*).

Emotional abuse This might be one person shouting constantly at the other, belittling her, or keeping her isolated. It may result in the victim of abuse being quiet and withdrawn.

Financial abuse If you notice any financial irregularities or theft from the person you are caring for, inform your supervisor. Keep receipts for goods that you buy on behalf of the person so that your conduct is beyond reproach.

HOW TO TREAT THE CARED FOR

The way you treat the person you are caring for will affect how she feels about herself. It is important that you respect her needs and that she trusts you. If respect and trust are established early on, you should be able to form a mutually beneficial relationship.

RESPECT THE INDIVIDUAL

When caring for someone, treat her with the utmost respect. Ask yourself how you would like to be treated, and make this the basis for the standard of care that you want to achieve. Find out as much as you can about the person you are caring for, and respect her individual needs. She may, for example, have specific dietary needs (*see page 64*), or be of a different sexual orientation or a different culture (*see page 37*). Never forget that she is an individual in her own right, and she is entitled to know what is happening to her. If there are changes to the care orders, explain them to her and, if possible, involve her in any decisions.

MAINTAIN CONFIDENTIALITY

It is important that the person you are caring for trusts you. To achieve this trust, you should respect her privacy and maintain confidentiality at all times. You have a duty to keep any information you may learn in your caregiving role confidential, including anything contained in the person's care records. The only exception to this is if you suspect abuse of any kind (*see left*); report this to your supervisor immediately, but do not discuss it with anyone else.

ADDRESSING PROBLEMS

At first you may not feel at ease with the person you are caring for, but, over time, you may be able to develop a good relationship. In some circumstances, however, you may be completely incompatible with the person, to the point where you cannot carry out care duties effectively. If these differences cannot be resolved, ask to be removed from that particular case. Remember, however, to strive for professionalism, even when you cannot communicate effectively with the person you are caring for.

CHAPTER 3

COMMUNICATION

Talking and listening to one another are essential
human needs. People need to communicate in order to express
their anxieties and emotions, and to make their wishes known.
Keeping the communication channels open when caring for your
relative can be beneficial to both of you, and it is important to
know what to do when communication becomes difficult.

COMMUNICATION SKILLS

Most human beings take verbal communication
for granted – so much so that they may not always bother to
make time for conversation. When you are caring for your relative,
making the time to talk and listen can enhance your
relationship and help iron out any difficulties.
You may be caring for someone with impaired
senses for whom verbal communication may be impossible; in
such a situation you may need to rely on nonverbal
skills, such as reading his body language and thinking about
how you use your own. Do not, for example, be
afraid to use touch, which can be reassuring as well as being
an effective way of conveying your feelings. You will also
need to explore ways in which you can help your
relative improve his communication skills.
This may be achieved by seeking specialist help and finding
out if there are any aids available that cater to your
relative's particular needs.

TALKING AND LISTENING

FINDING TIME FOR CONVERSATION is very important, especially to someone who is homebound or does not have contact with many people. It is easy to find excuses not to talk or listen, but if you make the time you may feel closer to the person for whom you are caring. Proper communication will allow both of you to express your feelings and help prevent resentment.

DO'S & DON'TS

☑ **Do** try to think about the way you are speaking and how your voice sounds. The pitch, rate, and rhythm of your voice are important if your relative has impaired hearing (*see page 41*).

☑ **Do** be patient if your relative has impaired speech (*see page 39*). Give him time to finish his sentence and resist the temptation to interrupt or speak for him.

☒ **Don't** patronize your relative. Whatever his disability, he should be treated with respect and not be addressed as if he were a child. A person who is physically impaired is still likely to be mentally alert.

☒ **Don't** exclude your relative from group conversations, whatever his condition. It may make him feel isolated and worthless if he is left alone in a corner watching and listening to other people talking.

IMPROVING COMMUNICATION

There are many reasons why communication can break down, making it difficult for you and your relative to talk to each other. It is important to keep the lines of communication open and to address any problems as early as possible.

MAKE TIME TO TALK

If you and your relative spend long periods of time together, you may become so familiar with each other that you do not notice hours passing without conversation. Also, as a caregiver, you will probably be extremely busy, and it may seem like a luxury to sit down and talk. But try not to think of it like that; allocate time to talk, even if it is only over a cup of coffee or between television programs. It could mean a great deal to your relative.

FIND COMMON INTERESTS

If your own lifestyle is restricted, it may be difficult to find things to talk about. However, it is usually possible to find subjects of mutual interest, such as sports, gardening, or television. Do not be afraid to talk about yourself and your interests. If your friends visit, try to include your relative in the discussions.

BE PATIENT

If your relative suffers from confusion or has impaired speech or hearing, verbal communication can be difficult and frustrating. You may sometimes feel that your patience is being pushed to the limit. Instead of getting angry, try taking deep breaths to calm yourself down or, after making sure that your relative is safe, leave the room for a few minutes until you are feeling less wound up.

THE VOLUNTEER CAREGIVER

W HEN YOU ARE A CAREGIVER from outside the home, it is essential to communicate effectively both with the person you are looking after and with the home caregiver, if there is one. This may range from the simple matter of being courteous, to overcoming language or cultural differences. Finding out as much as possible about the person you are caring for will help.

LANGUAGE AND CULTURAL DIFFERENCES

If the person you are caring for speaks a different language, communication can be difficult, but over time it should become easier. Be aware of any different cultural beliefs, and respect the fact that he may want to do things in a different way.

USE AN INTERPRETER
You may find that younger members of the family speak fluent English. Communicate either through one of them or ask your supervisor to arrange for an interpreter to accompany you, at least initially.

OBTAIN BILINGUAL MATERIAL
You can obtain information about relevant bilingual material, such as books and leaflets, from your library or the National Institutes of Health.

EDUCATE YOURSELF
Find out as much as possible about the person's beliefs by speaking to him or his family, and by obtaining information from your supervisor or local authority.

RESPECT THE PERSON'S WISHES
Beliefs and traditions may affect someone's lifestyle; this could include dietary restrictions (*see page 65*) or a woman not being allowed to be seen by a male doctor.

BE AWARE OF ISOLATION
Some members of ethnic minorities may have no contacts outside their immediate family, which can lead to a feeling of isolation. Discuss this problem with the affected person and his family, and try to find local activities that enable him to meet people who share his beliefs and interests.

RELATING TO THE HOME CAREGIVER

If there is already a home caregiver, she may resent your presence or even see it as an intrusion. Reassure her that you are there to support her, not to take over. Work with her to identify ways in which you can help.

Advice and support
You may be able to help with practical problems and, if she asks for it, give advice on the benefits and resources that are available to her.

Companionship The home caregiver may not come into contact with many people, so she may welcome a friendly face and the chance to talk to someone else.

Level of care If you and the home caregiver communicate well with one another and work together, the overall level of care given should improve, which will be beneficial to the person who is being cared for.

USING BODY LANGUAGE

A LTHOUGH MOST OF US express ourselves through the spoken word, we also communicate in many nonverbal ways. When you are caring for your relative, it will help if you understand his body language and know how to use your own. Body language is even more important if your relative's speech and hearing are impaired, rendering him unable to communicate verbally.

SIGNS OF ABUSE

You may suspect from your relative's body language that he is the victim of physical or emotional abuse. Abuse can take place in the home, as well as when the person is being cared for elsewhere. If you suspect abuse of any kind (see page 34), alert a care professional, but do not tell anyone else of your suspicions. Watch for behavioral changes or signs of injury.

Withdrawal The abused may isolate himself. He may appear wary of people and withdraw when he is approached.

Depression He may appear depressed or unusually quiet and avoid communication, especially eye contact.

Injury The abused may try to cover up bruising or other injuries. He may give unlikely explanations for how he has sustained his injuries.

THE PERSON BEING CARED FOR

Learning to read body language will help you care more effectively for your relative.

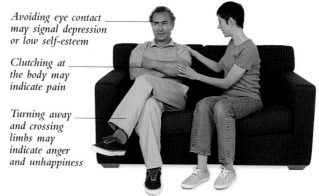

Avoiding eye contact may signal depression or low self-esteem

Clutching at the body may indicate pain

Turning away and crossing limbs may indicate anger and unhappiness

THE CAREGIVER

You can use your body language to help your relative feel more secure, thereby improving communication.

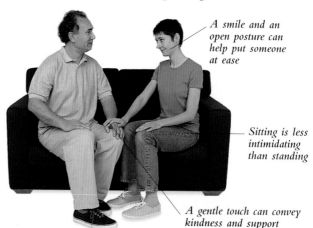

A smile and an open posture can help put someone at ease

Sitting is less intimidating than standing

A gentle touch can convey kindness and support

ADAPTING FOR SPECIAL NEEDS

COMMUNICATION DIFFICULTIES may arise when you are caring for someone with impaired speech, sight, or hearing. It is possible to overcome these difficulties by adapting the way in which you communicate. Many aids are available to help someone who has impaired senses to improve his ability to communicate and encourage independence.

IMPAIRED SPEECH

Helping someone to relearn how to speak can take a long time and requires a great deal of perseverance, patience, and encouragement. Talk to your relative's physician to find out what specialist help is available.

REASONS FOR SPEECH LOSS

There are a variety of possible reasons for speech loss or impairment of the voice.

Stroke The loss of speech that can occur after a stroke will be sudden. Your relative may know what he wants but be unable to communicate his needs, which can be very distressing. Often, he will literally have to be taught to speak again.

Voice box removal Someone who has had his voice box (*larynx*) removed will be more prepared for loss of speech. He may have a special device fitted that enables him to speak by modifying the sound produced by belching air from his stomach. This relearning process takes time and requires patience.

Brain damage Someone who is brain-damaged may be able to speak but be unable to find the right word. This can be frustrating for both of you, but with patience you can learn to understand his needs.

GETTING SPECIALIST HELP

You may, in time, learn to recognize what your relative is trying to say, but it will help both of you if you seek the help of a specialist.

Ask to see a speech–language pathologist
A physician can refer your relative to a speech-language pathologist, who is trained to recognize speech problems and to know how to overcome them. He will be able to help your relative with exercises, such as how to shape the mouth to form different sounds.

INDEPENDENCE AIDS

A person with impaired speech will be helped by having one or more of the items below to hand.

Pencil and paper
These should always be readily available so that your relative can write down requests.

Typing aids Specialized machines are available, or your relative could use a computer or typewriter in order to communicate his needs.

Visual aids He could hold up or point to images of frequently used items.

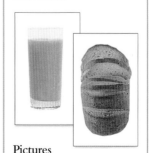

Pictures
Stick images from magazines onto cards.

INDEPENDENCE AIDS

Being registered blind (by an ophthalmologist) can make your relative eligible for a range of special services and equipment. Contact the American Council of the Blind (*see page 175*) for information. Your relative should find out from his physician what is available on prescription.

Telling the time Some clocks and watches have raised dots.

Playing games Modified sets of popular games are available.

Reading and writing Braille is a system of raised dots that is read by touch. Audiocassettes and large-print text also provide access to books.

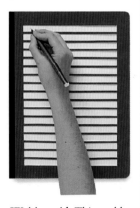

Writing aid This enables a visually impaired person to write in straight lines.

IMPAIRED SIGHT

This may be a condition present since birth, or it may come about as the result of disease or injury. If your relative's loss of sight is sudden, caused, perhaps, by an accident, it may be very frightening for him. If it develops gradually, you will both have time to get used to it and make the necessary adjustments. Try to help your relative maintain his independence wherever possible. (*See also page 76.*)

TYPES OF SIGHT LOSS

The level of impairment varies from person to person; few people have a complete lack of vision. Understanding the type of sight loss can enable you to help your relative. For instance, he may:

♦ distinguish only light
♦ have no central vision
♦ have no side vision
♦ see only a vague blur
♦ see only a mixture of blank spaces and defined areas.

COMMUNICATING WITH EACH OTHER

It is essential that your relative is independent and feels at ease in his home. The way you communicate with him is very important and may require you to adapt the way you would normally speak or respond.
Nonverbal signs Avoid responding nonverbally by nodding or shaking your head. Also, remember that body language, such as a smile or an outstretched hand, may be impossible for your relative to see.
Greetings and farewells When you approach a blind person, always say "Hello" and take his hand to shake it or pat his arm or shoulder to reassure him. If you do not know him well, identify yourself. Tell him when you are leaving so he is not left talking to himself.
Talking Do not change the way you speak. Do not be afraid to say "Nice to see you" – most blind people use this phrase themselves. If other people are nearby, address him by name or use a light touch on the arm to indicate that you are speaking to him.
Personal space To allow your relative maximum independence in the home, make sure his belongings and the items he frequently uses are kept in the same place; this will make it easier for him to locate things.

IMPAIRED HEARING

It is quite common for an elderly person's hearing to fail gradually. He may not realize that he is becoming deaf, or he may even refuse to accept his condition. Deafness may lead to feelings of isolation and rejection, and the person may think that people are talking about him or laughing at him behind his back. Try to be patient and reassuring.

COMMUNICATING WITH ONE ANOTHER

By reassessing the way in which you speak as well as the implications of your body language, you should be able to overcome the difficulties involved in communicating effectively.

Facing someone When you are talking to someone with impaired hearing, always face him so that he can lip-read what you are saying.

Tone of voice Learn to use the lower tones of your voice range because someone with impaired hearing is more able to hear these.

Body language Use nonverbal communication as much as possible. Your body language (*see page 38*) may be an essential way of communicating with someone whose hearing is impaired.

Sign language If your relative is deaf, it is useful to learn sign language. You could also develop your own signs between you.

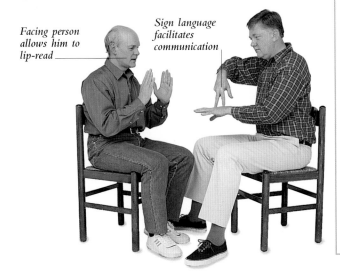

Facing person allows him to lip-read

Sign language facilitates communication

> ## INDEPENDENCE AIDS
>
> There is a range of aids available to help those with impaired hearing; information about these can be obtained from the National Association of the Deaf (*see page 175*). Before purchasing any aids, your relative should talk to his physician about the various types of hearing aids available and which is most suitable.
>
> **Hearing aid** In order to ensure that the hearing aid fits properly, a mold of your relative's ear will be taken. He should be warned that a hearing aid will magnify all sounds equally, to prepare him for this when he is in particularly noisy places. In order to work effectively, the hearing aid should not get wet, and the batteries should be checked regularly.
>
> **Specialized telephones** A variety of telephones are available; a flashing light can indicate ringing and some display the message on a screen.
>
> **Amplifying sound** Personal amplifiers such as earphones increase the sound of a television or radio. Portable amplifiers can be attached to the earpiece of a telephone.

DEALING WITH CONFUSION

I F A PERSON IS CONFUSED, he may forget simple facts, such as what day of the week it is, who someone is, or his own whereabouts. This can be frustrating for both of you and potentially dangerous for your relative. Although looking after a confused person requires patience, there are some practical steps you can take to help him remember things and become less dependent on you.

SHORT-TERM CONFUSION

Confusion is not always a long-term problem. It is often a temporary condition, most common when the person is ill.

Due to illness
Sometimes an acute infection, for example, can cause temporary confusion. Give your relative plenty of fluids to prevent him from becoming dehydrated and to help lessen the confusion. Consult the physician or nurse practioner for advice.

Drug-related
Both confusion and behavioral changes may coincide with your relative being put on new medication. If this occurs, inform his physician of the problem so that a change of medication or dosage can be considered. Drug-related confusion can also occur when a person has taken a medication for a long time.

MEMORY LOSS

Confusion can cause or be the result of memory loss. Someone who has lost the ability to add to his long-term memory may forget something you said ten seconds ago, but be able to remember clearly an event that happened ten years ago. He may ask you the same question over and over again; not only has he forgotten the answer, he has probably forgotten that he ever asked you the question.

COMMUNICATING INFORMATION
You can help your relative by thinking about the way you communicate information.
Use active phrases Say, "It is time to take your tablets." Do not tell him hours before, "You need to take your tablets at three o'clock."
Be specific Be precise when writing a reminder: "Your hospital appointment is at 11am on Thursday, May 16th," not "Hospital appointment, Thursday."
Keep questions direct Ask your relative, "Would you like tea or coffee?" Do not ask him, "What would you like to drink?"

INDEPENDENCE AIDS
Use some of the methods recommended below to encourage independence. Discuss these with your relative first because he may resent the house being cluttered with reminders telling him what to do.
Clocks and calendars All clocks and calendars should be correct; an alarm clock could be set for the time your relative needs to take his medication.
Notice board List the things that are happening that day, such as visitors expected or outings planned.
Notes Place reminder notes, such as "Have you turned the oven off?" in strategic places.

CHAPTER 4

ADAPTING THE HOME

One of the main aims of caregiving is to help your relative maintain independence. To achieve this, it may be necessary to make some changes to the home environment. This chapter includes ideas for adapting every room in the home and outlines the range of benefits that may be available to enable you to do this. For example, if your relative uses a wheelchair and home alterations are necessary in order to accommodate it, you may be able to obtain a mortgage to cover the expense.

WHAT YOU CAN DO

Adaptations should always be safe and, wherever possible, also suitable for able-bodied members of the household. Simple measures, such as rearranging furniture and moving unnecessary clutter out of the way, can create space and allow someone to move around more easily; giving thought to where frequently needed items are placed can enable your relative to do more for herself. If she has mobility problems or is confined to a wheelchair, it may be necessary to obtain specialized equipment or make structural changes, such as widening doors. It is essential that you discuss any changes with your relative beforehand and that she is happy with them; otherwise, it could be confusing for her to find things rearranged, especially if she has been in the hospital a long time.

GETTING HELP

ALWAYS SEEK THE ADVICE of an occupational therapist before embarking on any adaptations or purchasing specialized equipment. An occupational therapist is trained to assess the needs of the person you are caring for and advise on possible funding. A special grant or loan may be available if it is essential to purchase specialized equipment and/or make structural changes.

CASE STUDY

NAME: DOROTHY
AGE: 56

Dorothy, who is wheelchair bound due to a spinal injury, wanted to continue living in her apartment. To make this feasible, she obtained funding to make major adaptations to her kitchen and bathroom. However, some relatively minor problems still bothered her: for example, she couldn't get clothes out of the closet or reach outlets. She contacted a volunteer organization, who was able to arrange for additional changes to be made, including moving door handles to the hinge side of the door (so she would not have to lean too far out of her wheelchair to open it), lowering closet rods, and raising outlets. These small changes enabled Dorothy to be more independent in her own home and helped improve her quality of life.

MAKING THE RIGHT ADAPTATIONS

Obtaining the right advice before you begin adapting the home is essential to your relative's safety and your own, and it can prevent you from wasting time and money making changes that are of limited use. The Americans with Disabilities Act (1990) required newly built public buildings to be accessible to people with physical disabilities, and existing buildings to be adapted if it could be done without significant expense. Many changes made to public buildings have been adapted for use in private homes.

ECHO HOUSING

Elder Cottage Housing Opportunity, more commonly known as ECHO housing, provides an opportunity for your relative to live near you without moving into your house. If the local zoning regulations allow it, ECHO houses can be built on your property. These one-story units consist of living and eating areas, a bedroom, a kitchen, and a bathroom, all specifically designed for your relative's needs. Most houses can be removed and resold when they are no longer needed.

MAKING SHORT-TERM CHANGES

In some circumstances, ECHO housing or permanent changes on your own house may be unnecessary. Your relative may be convalescing after an illness and her mobility, for example, may be affected for only a short amount of time. In this situation, look for practical and inexpensive ways to adapt your home. For instance, instead of putting up an extra banister, would it be possible for your relative to sleep downstairs for a few weeks? If your relative needs specialized equipment for only a short time, could you borrow it from a volunteer organization?

GETTING FINANCIAL HELP

Your local or state housing authority will be able to tell you whether you and your relative are eligible for financial benefits to meet the cost of purchasing specialized equipment or making essential structural changes, and if such programs are available in your area. State finance agencies, departments of public welfare, community development departments, and building inspection departments may also provide information. Make sure that you have investigated all the possible public sources of funding before pursuing private sources.

PUBLIC SOURCES OF FUNDING

Funds may be obtained from a variety of public sources. The following three are the most common, but others may also be worth investigation; be sure to research all available options thoroughly.
The Farmers Home Administration (FmHA) provides loans, as well as grants to low-income prople over 62, for home alterations and repair in rural areas.
Department of Housing and Urban Development (HUD) distributes a variety of loans, including the Community Development Block program. These funds are administered by the local government, which, in some cases, designates some of the money to be used by elderly people to fix their homes.
The Veterans Administration (VA) may provide low-interest loans to veterans who need to make their homes more accessible.
What amount of funding will be provided? This will depend on your relative's income and ability to pay.
How do I/we apply? You or your relative should write to the appropriate agency. Be sure to include in your request for funds the medical problem and your proposed solution, the total cost, and the amount you are able to pay. Medical documentation and an itemized cost estimate are often helpful.

MINOR WORK

Some volunteer organizations will do minor changes, such as installing an access ramp into the house, or necessary home maintenance, including painting, to enable the person to remain in familiar surroundings.

BUYING EQUIPMENT

Most equipment and supplies can be obtained through mail-order companies or from a medical equipment company, or a pharmacist may be able to order it. They can also be rented or bought through a home care agency. Seek advice on the installation and use of all equipment.

Testing equipment
When purchasing expensive equipment, visit a Disabled Living Center to examine and test the items on display. Manufacturers may come to your home to demonstrate very specialized equipment.

Second-hand equipment Many volunteer organizations provide used medical equipment. If acquiring second-hand equipment, use more caution than for new products.

Taxes Any equipment, necessary furniture, and permanent changes to the house are deductible from federal income tax as medical expenses. Call the local Internal Revenue Service office or a tax consultant for up-to-date information and filing requirements.

GENERAL IMPROVEMENTS

I<small>F A PERSON IS SICK OR HAS LIMITED MOBILITY,</small> her quality of life may be
greatly improved if she can get around the home easily and do things by
herself. For example, simply rearranging furniture may be all she needs to be
able to walk around safely and without your assistance. Look around your
home for anything that could possibly pose a hazard for your relative.

ADAPTATIONS AROUND THE HOME

For general safety, don't leave items
lying around on the floor. Tape down
anything, such as electrical cords, that
is likely to trip up your relative.
Floors Remove rugs or secure to the
floor with double-sided tape. Choose
plain floors if your relative can't see well.
Windows and curtains For those
who are unable to stretch, long-handled
openers for windows, and curtains with
pulleys, are recommended. Electrically
operated devices are also available.

Plugs and outlets Plugs with handles
are useful for those with limited
dexterity. Position outlets higher up
on the wall for a wheelchair user.
Communication aids Intercom
systems enable an immobile person
to find out who is at the door and to
communicate from another room. A
panic button, attached to a help point,
can be installed. This service is available
from many sources, including medical
suppliers; ask your physician for advice.

IMPROVING ACCESS INTO AND OUT OF THE HOME

Determine how easy it is for your
relative to enter and leave the home,
and make improvements, if possible.

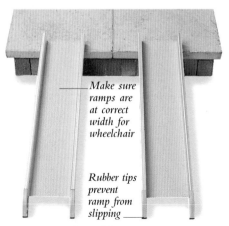

*Make sure
ramps are
at correct
width for
wheelchair*

*Rubber tips
prevent
ramp from
slipping*

Portable ramps

Gates or doors It may be necessary
to widen gates or doors for wheelchair
access – a width of 32in (80cm) is the
minimum advised, but 40in (100cm) is
preferable. Remove door sills, if possible,
since these can be hazardous and impede
people who are confined to wheelchairs,
and those who use walking aids.
Garden access Paths should be level or
have only gentle slopes and be nonslip.
They may need to be widened if
wheelchair access is necessary. Also, don't
put gravel down because this can make
it difficult to push a wheelchair.
Ramps These can be installed over
single steps to facilitate wheelchair
access. You can get permanent ones or
lightweight portable ones to make it
easier to get into and out of the house.

HALLWAY AND STAIRS

THE MOST IMPORTANT OBSTRUCTIONS for your relative in her attempt to move around the house may be found in the hallway and on the stairs. Hallways should be adapted to suit your relative's disability. Extra rails, or even a stairlift, can make all the difference to a disabled person who can't otherwise get up and down the stairs, and enable her to lead as normal a life as possible.

ADAPTING THE HALLWAY

Make sure that nothing in the hallway is preventing your relative from moving around easily.

Lighting levels The hallway, landing, and stairs should be well lit, especially for someone with impaired sight.

Furniture If your relative uses a wheelchair or walker around the house, keep the hallway as clear of furniture as possible. However, for someone who is unsteady on her feet, heavy furniture in the hall may be useful as a support.

Grab rails Place these at appropriate places along the wall to help an unsteady person walk down the hall.

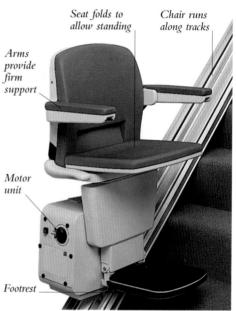

Seat folds to allow standing

Chair runs along tracks

Arms provide firm support

Motor unit

Footrest

Grab rail

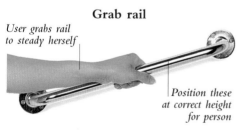

User grabs rail to steady herself

Position these at correct height for person

ADAPTING THE STAIRS

This may involve installing an extra banister or, more expensively, a stairlift.

Stairgate A gate at the top and bottom of the stairs may help if the person suffers from confusion.

Banisters An extra banister placed along the wall makes it much easier for a person to get up or down stairs.

Stairlift A person who has difficulty climbing the stairs, or who is wheelchair bound, will benefit from the use of a stairlift. This is a seat attached to the staircase. The person sits in it and presses a button; it then moves slowly up or down the staircase.

Vertical through-floor elevator This elevator is installed in a first-floor room. The person is transported through a "trapdoor" in the ceiling to a room upstairs. It is very useful for wheelchair users who need a wheelchair upstairs, or where a stairlift cannot be fitted.

KITCHEN

TO BE ABLE TO COOK BY HERSELF, your relative should have all the necessary kitchen facilities. This will reduce the burden on you, the caregiver, if you are the only person preparing meals. In addition to making structural changes, you may need to obtain eating and drinking aids to help her to eat and drink by herself as well as to cook and prepare food (*see page 68*).

ADAPTING THE KITCHEN

Consider simple changes, such as having an eating area in the kitchen so that your relative does not have to carry hot food to another room. Check that seating is comfortable and safe; a chair with arms is more suitable than a stool. If structural changes are necessary, opt for adaptations that will also suit other, able-bodied members of the household.

Adjustable sink height

Cart to transport hot items

High oven is ideal for someone who can't bend

Lighting Strip lighting placed under wall units and shelves is especially useful for someone with impaired sight.
Cabinets and drawers Choose units with drawers that can be pulled straight out so that all items can be accessed easily. Specialized cabinets with shelves that pull out farther are also available. If ordinary drawers and cabinets are being used, make sure frequently used items are easy to find and reach.
Work surfaces If possible, fit pull-out work surfaces that are the correct height for a wheelchair user.
Stoves and ovens Control knobs should be positioned at the front of the stove to allow your relative to operate the oven without having to stretch over the hot stove. When you or your relative is cooking, be sure that the handles of any pans or skillets are turned toward the middle of the stove to reduce the chance of burns or scalds. Pot-holders or oven mitts should be obvious and positioned low enough that a wheelchair user can reach them easily and quickly when necessary.

LIVING ROOM

T HIS MAY BE THE ROOM where an inactive person spends most of her time. It should be made as comfortable as possible so that she can enjoy her leisure time independently. It is important to get the right type of chair for her to sit in: one that she is comfortable in and that she can get into and out of fairly easily. Make sure that everything she needs is within easy reach.

ADAPTING THE LIVING ROOM

If your relative has mobility problems, she should be seated in the best position in the room. Ideally, sit her by the window so that she can see outside, but ensure that she is shaded from direct sunlight.

Footrest This can provide comfort for someone who is seated. A bean bag is an ideal footrest.

Remote control systems Get your relative a television or stereo that has a remote control so that she is able to operate it from her chair. Those who have very limited mobility can even get remote-controlled curtains and lights.

BUYING A CHAIR

If you are purchasing a chair for someone who is weak or immobile, choose one that has firm arms and a high seat so it is easier for her to get into and out of by herself. Alternatively, there is a variety of specialized chairs that can be self-operated to raise the user to a standing position.

Mechanical chair

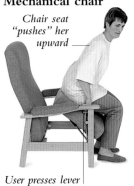

Chair seat "pushes" her upward

User presses lever

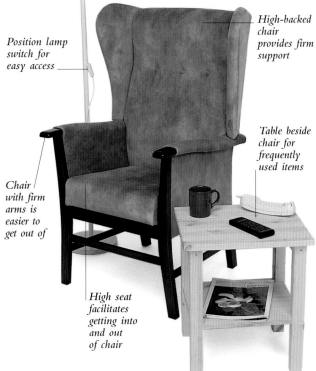

Position lamp switch for easy access

Chair with firm arms is easier to get out of

High-backed chair provides firm support

Table beside chair for frequently used items

High seat facilitates getting into and out of chair

BATHROOM AND TOILET

I F YOUR RELATIVE NEEDS YOUR HELP to wash and to use the toilet, it may be embarrassing for her and time-consuming for you. It may help to get the bathroom and toilet altered so that she can use them by herself. It is also worth considering how difficult it is for her to reach the bathroom and toilet, and, if possible, making the route easier. (*See also* Personal Care, *pages 97–106.*)

ADAPTING THE BATHROOM AND TOILET

Some alterations to the layout of the bathroom and toilet are essential for safety. An ideal layout is shown below, but you may find that a rail or a frame around the toilet is all that is necessary.
Bathroom or toilet door Sliding or folding doors allow easier wheelchair

access and may also make it easier for you to reach a person who has fallen.
Floor Wall-to-wall carpet is safer than a tiled or linoleum floor, which can be slippery when wet.
Frames or grab rails Fitted around the toilet, bathtub, or shower, these can provide enough support to allow a weak person to use the bathroom alone.

TOILET SEAT

The toilet seat can be raised to help a weak person get on and off it more easily. This can be done by installing a base under the toilet or by fitting an elevated toilet seat. These seats fit on most standard toilets and are removable so that they can be washed.

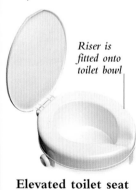

Riser is fitted onto toilet bowl

Elevated toilet seat

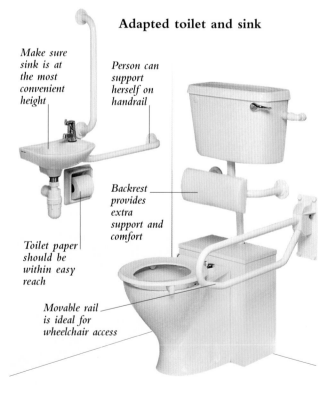

Adapted toilet and sink

Make sure sink is at the most convenient height

Person can support herself on handrail

Backrest provides extra support and comfort

Toilet paper should be within easy reach

Movable rail is ideal for wheelchair access

SINKS

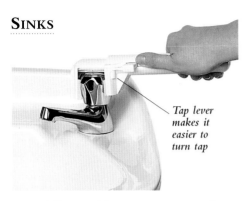

Tap lever makes it easier to turn tap

Taps Those with cross tops are easier to operate than rounded ones, which can be difficult to grip. You can install replacement lever taps, or fit temporary levers. These enable a person with weak hands or wrists to turn the tap on and off with ease.

Sink height Sinks may need to be lowered for a wheelchair user or raised for a person who cannot bend easily.

BATHS AND SHOWERS

To enable your relative to wash herself, you may need to adapt your bathtub or shower. Place a mat inside and beside the bathtub to prevent accidents. Avoid using bath oils since they can make the tub slippery.

Bath seat This can be placed in the bathtub when your relative wants to use it *(see page 98)*. Mechanical seats called "bath-lifters," which can be self-operated, are also available.

Showerstall If a person has difficulty getting into a bathtub, a showerstall is often a simpler option. Shower units with level or ramped access, instead of sills that have to be stepped or wheeled over, are much easier to use. Make sure that the shower has nonslip tiling, or use a mat.

Shower seat This can be placed in the showerstall and is useful fore someone who is too weak to stand. A chair that can be wheeled into the shower is also available, but door sills may have to be removed if this is used.

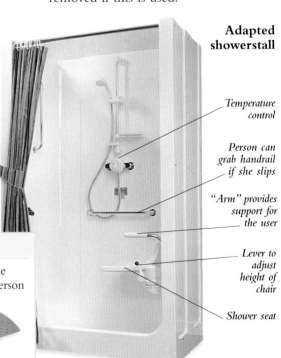

Adapted showerstall

Temperature control

Person can grab handrail if she slips

"Arm" provides support for the user

Lever to adjust height of chair

Shower seat

NONSLIP MATS

A nonslip mat should be placed in the bathtub or showerstall to prevent a person from slipping when she gets in and out.

Pads on bottom grip surface

BEDROOM

IF THE MAJORITY OF PRACTICAL CARE is carried out in this room, there must be sufficient space around the bed to carry out procedures safely and easily. It may also be necessary to raise a low bed. If your relative can get out of bed but has mobility problems, you may need to adapt her closet so that she can get her clothes more easily. (*See also* Bed Comfort, *pages 83–96*.)

ADAPTING THE BEDROOM

This room should be comfortable and easy to use, especially for someone who is confined to bed for long periods. Light switches and lamps should be near the bed – select an angled lamp if the person likes to read in bed. If a toilet aid is used (*see page 114*), keep it near the bed. Place a suitable chair, with armrests and a firm seat, next to the bed for your relative to sit in.
Cabinet doors and shelving Closets with sliding doors and pull-out shelves enable someone who has difficulty stretching to reach clothes.

Closets Lowering rods and handles helps a wheelchair user to reach clothes.
Television and radio Obtain equipment that has a remote control.

BED RISERS

These can be attached to the legs of a low bed to raise it so the person can get in and out easily (the bed should be no lower than knee-high), and to minimize any risk of back strain to you. Ask a healthcare professional which type should be used.

Bed leg

Castor fits tightly in hole

Circular base rests flat on floor

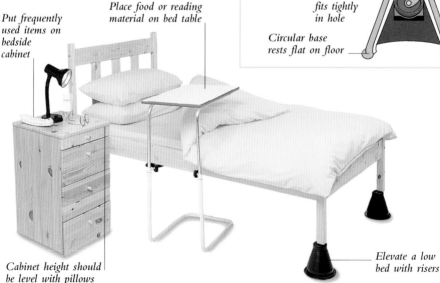

Put frequently used items on bedside cabinet

Place food or reading material on bed table

Cabinet height should be level with pillows

Elevate a low bed with risers

CHAPTER 5

HOME HYGIENE

If your relative is sick or frail, or is taking certain
types of medications, he may be particularly vulnerable
to infection, so it is essential to maintain as hygienic and
germfree an environment as possible. It is also important to
protect yourself from infection because if you get sick, not only
will you be unable to fulfill your role efficiently, you may
also put your relative's health at risk.

CLEANLINESS

There are many preventive measures you can take
to eliminate germs (such as *bacteria* and *viruses*) and minimize
the spread of infection. The most important of these measures is
to maintain a high standard of personal hygiene: a simple task
such as handwashing is often done in a quick, perfunctory
way, but washing your hands thoroughly is an essential
part of basic cleanliness.

DISPOSAL OF WASTE

If your relative is sick or incontinent, part of your
caregiving role may include dealing with the disposal of his body
waste, such as blood, vomit, feces, or urine.
It is essential that you follow the correct procedures for the
disposal of this waste to minimize the risk of infecting
yourself and to prevent any infection from
spreading to other people.

INFECTION AND ITS CAUSES

AN INFECTION IS THE RESULT of the body being invaded by germs (such as *bacteria* and *viruses*). This causes an adverse reaction – directly by damaging cells, or indirectly by releasing poisonous substances (*toxins*) into the body. The symptoms will depend on the type of infection, where it is located, and whether it has spread throughout the body.

THE SYMPTOMS OF INFECTION

The symptoms of an infection depend on whether the infection is confined to one area or has spread throughout the body (*see opposite* and *pages 178–80*). For example, an infection caused by an abscess may be localized, whereas the infection caused by chickenpox, measles, or a common cold will affect the whole body.

Symptoms of a localized infection may be:
◆ pain and swelling
◆ localized redness
◆ loss of movement
◆ areas that are hot to the touch.

Symptoms of an infection throughout the body may be:
◆ raised temperature and increased breathing and pulse rates (*see page 128*)
◆ headache and thirst
◆ hot, dry skin, and rash
◆ loss of appetite
◆ weakness and apathy.

HOW INFECTION SPREADS

An infection is only dangerous if it is given a suitable environment in which to flourish.

Sources People and animals are the sources of most infections, carrying many bacteria and viruses.

Routes An infection can be contracted through direct and indirect routes (*see below*).

Victim Anyone can become infected, but the most vulnerable are those who have not been vaccinated and those who have low immunity (*see page 56*), such as a frail person or someone in poor health.

DIRECT AND INDIRECT ROUTES

A person can catch an infection *directly* by touching something that is contaminated; by sharing a needle with a contaminated person; through an exchange of body fluids such as blood or saliva; or through sexual activity with an infected person. An infection can be spread *indirectly* in a variety of ways.

Airborne Germs can be carried in the droplets of fluid expelled when coughing and sneezing.

Food Contamination can result if food is not stored, handled, or cooked correctly (*see page 60*).

Clothing or equipment These can harbor germs if they are not cleaned regularly and thoroughly.

Insects A number of insects, especially houseflies, can spread infection.

TREATING INFECTION

If you think you or your relative has an infection, seek medical help as soon as possible. The physician may prescribe a course of antibiotics for bacterial infections; these will be effective only if the course is completed. If the infection is viral, the physician will usually only be able to treat the symptoms.

Some Infectious Diseases (see also pages 178–80)

Disease	Possible Signs and Symptoms	How it may be Transmitted	Infectious Period
Gastro-enteritis	Appetite loss, nausea, vomiting, diarrhea, abdominal cramps.	Contaminated food or water supplies.	Up to two days after diarrhea stops.
Infectious mononu-cleosis	Fever, headache, swollen glands in neck, armpits, and groin, severe sore throat, fatigue.	Contact with saliva.	Variable – may be weeks.
Hepatitis A, B, C, D and E	Flulike illness, followed by jaundice. Some people have no symptoms.	A, E: infected food or water; B, C, D: sexually transmitted; contaminated blood; shared needles.	A, E: one week after jaundice. B, C, D: varies; blood can be infectious for life.
Herpes simplex (cold sores and genital herpes)	Small, fluid-filled, irritating blisters, slight temperature.	Contact with lesions.	Until blisters have formed crusts.
Herpes zoster (chickenpox and shingles)	Chickenpox: slight fever, groups of itchy, dark red spots that become blisters. Shingles: localized, painful, blistering rash.	Airborne; contact with rash.	Until all blisters have formed scabs.
HIV/AIDS	May be symptomless for years; breathlessness, fever, weight loss, diarrhea, swollen glands, and fatigue may eventually occur.	Sexually transmitted; contaminated blood; shared needles; mother to child.	For life.
Influenza, common cold	Fever, cough, runny nose, headache, sore throat, chills, aches, pains.	Airborne.	First few days.
Meningitis	Fever, stiff neck, headache, drowsiness, confusion, rash, reaction to light.	Various methods, usually airborne.	A week before and ten days after fever.
Tuber-culosis	Fever, cough, swollen and painful glands, stiff neck, weight loss.	Airborne.	While phlegm is infected.

Preventing Infection

THE BODY'S IMMUNE SYSTEM cannot fully protect against infection. It is essential, therefore, for your own health and for that of your relative, to take steps to eliminate the germs that cause infection from your home environment. The risks can be minimized if you maintain a good level of cleanliness and take proper precautions when dealing with body waste.

Personal Hygiene

You can maintain a high standard of cleanliness and minimize the risk of infection by washing your hands thoroughly and wearing disposable gloves. It is important that you follow the correct technique for removing gloves once they are soiled.

The Body's Natural Defenses

The immune system is the body's main defense against infection. White blood cells circulate around the body and destroy harmful bacteria. People with leukemia, for example, who have a low number of these cells, are more prone to infection.

Washing Your Hands Thoroughly

Wash your hands before and after preparing food, after using the toilet, and before and after giving care, even if gloves are worn. Scrub dirty nails as part of your handwashing routine.

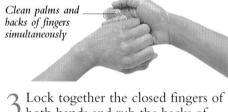

Clean palms and backs of fingers simultaneously

1 Wet and soap your hands. Rub your palms together to form a lather.

To clean thoroughly, build up rich lather

2 Rub the palm and fingers of one hand over the back of the other, interlocking the fingers. Repeat for the other hand.

Clean back of hand and between fingers

3 Lock together the closed fingers of both hands and rub the backs of them against your palms.

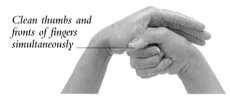

Clean thumbs and fronts of fingers simultaneously

4 Clean each thumb by rubbing it against the fronts of your fingers.

5 Clean your fingertips by rubbing them on the palm of the opposite hand. This also cleans the palm.

6 Rinse your hands and dry them on a clean cloth or paper towel.

WEARING AND REMOVING GLOVES

Gloves should be worn whenever a procedure involves contact with body fluids, and when creams or lotions are being applied. To prevent any substance from coming into contact with your skin, always remove gloves using the procedure below. Disposable latex or vinyl gloves are available from most pharmacies. The thinner polyethylene varieties should not be used since they do not provide adequate protection.

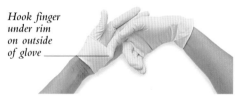

Hook finger under rim on outside of glove

1 Pick up the base of the left-hand glove with your right index finger. Pull it halfway off your hand, leaving the top half of your thumb covered.

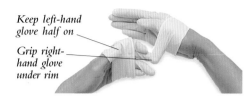

Keep left-hand glove half on

Grip right-hand glove under rim

2 Repeat step 1 to remove the glove on your right hand, but this time pull the glove all the way off, so that it is completely inside out.

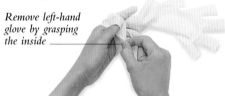

Remove left-hand glove by grasping the inside

3 Use your now uncovered right hand to pull the left glove off, so that both gloves are now inside out.

4 Pick up the gloves on the inside and dispose of them safely.

CLEANING EQUIPMENT

Some of the items used when caring may be disposable, but others will require thorough cleaning.
Toilet aids (*see page 114*) Clean bedpans, urinals, and commodes with hot, soapy water.
Thermometers (*see pages 126–28*) Before use, rinse the thermometer in cold water and dry it with a paper towel. After use, wipe it with a damp cloth or cotton.
Washing accessories Launder towels and washcloths regularly. It is advisable to use separate towels and washcloths on the body and face.
Surfaces Clean surfaces such as table-tops and bed-trays with a detergent, and dry thoroughly with a clean cloth.

CONTAINING YOUR OWN GERMS

It is particularly important to take steps to make sure that you do not spread your own germs to your relative.

Illness If you are sick, it will not help either you or your relative if you continue caregiving. Inform a care professional so that alternative arrangements can be made (*see pages 24–25*).

Coughing and sneezing Use a tissue or handkerchief and avoid coughing or sneezing in the direction of your relative.

Skin infections If you have cuts, abrasions, or a skin disorder, you must make sure that the entire area is properly protected by gloves or a waterproof dressing before giving care.

NEEDLE AND SYRINGE DISPOSAL

If a medication has to be given by injection, or if your relative has to test his blood through pin-pricks, the safe disposal of needles and syringes is essential. These should be placed in an American Standards Approved sharps disposal container, which is supplied by local health services and medical suppliers. A healthcare professional will arrange to collect and dispose of the box at regular agreed intervals. Follow these guidelines:

◆ keep the sharps box out of reach of children to prevent them from hurting themselves with the needles;

◆ do not fill the box more than three-quarters full;

◆ do not place the box in a domestic trash bag.

Sharps disposal container

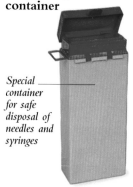

Special container for safe disposal of needles and syringes

DISPOSING OF BODY WASTE

When you are caring for someone, you should take precautions to prevent yourself and anyone else from coming into contact with that person's body waste. The risk of spreading infection can be greatly reduced if you take the necessary preventive measures. When disposing of waste, wear latex gloves and an apron, if available. If you are caring for someone suffering from a blood-borne infection, such as HIV or hepatitis, seek advice from the person's physician.

METHODS OF DISPOSAL

There are two safe ways to dispose of waste.
Down the toilet Place body fluids and soiled tissues in the toilet, close the lid, and flush the toilet twice.
In a plastic bag Some waste materials, such as dressings and incontinence pads, should be placed in a secure plastic bag, which must be sealed before being placed in the trash can – never flush these materials down the toilet. If your relative has a blood-borne infection, official yellow plastic bags will be supplied and collected for incineration.

CLEANING SPILLAGES

Wearing latex gloves, cover the body waste with paper towels and pour undiluted bleach over the towels if the waste is on a hard surface. Gather it all up with clean paper towels and dispose of it in a sealed plastic bag. If the spill is on a carpet, use hot, soapy water, not bleach.

NEEDLE INJURY

If you accidentally prick yourself with a used needle, or another sharp object that has come into contact with body fluids, do not suck the injury to stop it from bleeding. To prevent the spread of infection, follow this procedure:
◆ wash the affected area under cold, running water;

◆ encourage the wound to bleed freely;

◆ inform your physician or other healthcare professional.

If you are a volunteer caregiver, you must inform the organization for whom you are working so that the incident can be documented.

CHAPTER 6

HEALTHY EATING & DRINKING

Your relative may have a small appetite or find eating difficult because of an illness, a disability, or general apathy, but it is essential to encourage her to eat regularly and well. Achieving a balanced diet is always possible, even if someone has to follow a special diet for health or personal reasons. To help you meet the requirements of a balanced diet, this chapter provides a basic understanding of nutrition.

MAKING MEALTIMES ENJOYABLE

To make mealtimes enjoyable and relaxed, try to gain an understanding of your relative's needs and, if she is physically impaired, find practical ways that allow her to be more independent when eating or drinking. Simple measures can be taken to make meals look and taste as appetizing as possible; this is especially important for someone who is sick and does not have a strong appetite.

CARING FOR YOURSELF

As a caregiver it is easy to neglect your own needs and get into bad habits, such as skipping meals or snacking. To meet the high energy demands required for caregiving, however, it is essential that you also eat sensibly and regularly (*see page 19*).

HYGIENE IN THE KITCHEN

SOMEONE WHO IS SICK OR FRAIL may be particularly vulnerable to infection. It is, therefore, essential to take simple steps when preparing and cooking food to reduce the risk of contamination. In order to minimize any health risks, you need to keep your kitchen and cooking utensils clean, shop sensibly, store food wisely, and prepare it carefully.

DO'S & DON'TS

Follow these guidelines when you are buying and storing food:

☑ **Do** check that the inner wrapping of packaged foods, and the seals and rims of canned foods, are not damaged.

☑ **Do** check the expiration date on foods before purchasing them.

☑ **Do** put food in the refrigerator or freezer as soon as possible.

☑ **Do** place fruit and vegetables in the bottom of the refrigerator, and fish and meat in the coldest part. Clean these appliances regularly.

☒ **Don't** store raw and cooked foods on the same shelf. Put raw meat and defrosting products on a plate to keep them from dripping.

☒ **Don't** put raw and frozen foods in the same shopping bag. Put frozen food in an insulated bag, if you have one.

HYGIENE TIPS

To prevent food contamination, make the following simple steps part of your daily routine when using your kitchen and preparing and cooking meals.

CLEANLINESS
♦ Keep pets away from all food and kitchen surfaces.
♦ Wash your hands before and after preparing food.
♦ Clean utensils and cutting tools thoroughly.
♦ Change and launder towels and cloths regularly.
♦ Avoid wiping your hands repeatedly on an apron or cloth; do not use dishtowels as handtowels.
♦ Cover any cuts or sores on your hands.

PREPARATION
♦ Do not eat food from damaged containers, or food that has passed its expiration date.
♦ Wash fresh fruit and vegetables thoroughly.
♦ Do not use the same knife or chopping board to prepare cooked and uncooked foods at the same time.
♦ Do not prepare food too far in advance.
♦ Follow frozen food guidelines carefully.

COOKING
♦ Ensure that all meat and fish is thoroughly cooked.
♦ Do not taste food with your fingers.
♦ When reheating food, check that it is thoroughly hot and do not reheat it more than once.
♦ Follow cooking guidelines exactly on all products.
♦ Eat cooked food while it is hot.
♦ Avoid giving the following foods to the sick or elderly: pâté or soft cheeses, which may contain listeria bacteria; either raw or undercooked eggs, or undercooked meat, especially poultry, which can cause salmonella poisoning.

EATING A BALANCED DIET

To MAINTAIN GOOD HEALTH you need to eat the right balance of foods from each of the five main food groups (*see page 63*) and drink plenty of fluids. Provided that no particular food is eaten in excess and sufficient calories are consumed for the body's daily needs (2,750 calories for a physically active man, 2,000 for a physically active woman), your diet should be well balanced.

WHAT YOUR BODY NEEDS

Your body needs a combination of nutrients – proteins, carbohydrates, fats, vitamins, minerals, and fiber – to satisfy all of its requirements.

PROTEINS

Proteins supply the body with the amino acids that are required to build new protein. Animal foods provide all the essential amino acids, while plant foods need to be combined (*see page 64*).

CARBOHYDRATES

These are starches or sugars and are the body's main source of energy. Starches are broken down into single molecules by the digestive system before being absorbed into the bloodstream, and often contain beneficial fiber (*see below*). Sugars are absorbed rapidly, supplying an instant, but short-term, surge of energy.

FATS

These are a good energy source (especially for those who have high energy requirements, such as the elderly) and are an essential component of the body's cells. However, saturated fat in particular should be eaten in moderation due to the risk of heart disease and obesity.

VITAMINS AND MINERALS

These help the body function properly and contribute to overall good health. A balanced diet usually provides a sufficient quantity of each one.

FIBER

This passes through the body unchanged and is essential in preventing bowel and digestive problems. Fiber is also filling and therefore may reduce calorie intake.

FOOD SOURCES

Where to find the food types contained in a balanced diet.

Animal foods   Meat, poultry, fish, eggs, milk, and cheese.

Plant foods   Bread, pasta, potatoes, rice, beans, and pulses.

Starches   Potatoes, bread, rice, pasta, and some fruits.

Sugars   Table sugar, candy, cookies, and jam.

Unsaturated fats   Oily fish, some vegetable oils, and margarine.

Saturated fats   Red meat, whole milk and other dairy products.

Vitamins and minerals   Found in a variety of foods (*see pages 62–63*); a balanced diet should prevent the need for supplements.

Fiber   Wholemeal bread, cereals, potatoes, peas, bananas, oranges, and green vegetables.

WHAT VITAMINS CAN DO

VITAMIN	WHAT IT DOES	WHERE IT CAN BE FOUND
A	Necessary for normal growth and vision, protects against infection.	Liver, fish-liver oils, egg yolk, dairy products, margarine, oranges, carrots.
Vitamin B complex, including B_1, B_2, B_6	Promotes breakdown of fats, carbohydrates, and proteins. Helps form important body constituents, such as heart and body muscle.	Pasta, bran, wholemeal bread, meat, eggs, beans, cereals.
B_{12}	Helps to form red blood cells and to keep the nervous system healthy.	Offal, chicken, fish, eggs, dairy products.
C	Maintains healthy bones and teeth; aids iron absorption.	Vegetables, fruit, especially citrus fruit, potatoes.
D	Essential for strong bones and teeth; aids calcium absorption.	Oily fish, liver, milk, egg yolk, margarine; in skin from sunlight.
E	Aids formation of red blood cells; slows down cell aging.	Vegetable oils, nuts, meat, green vegetables, cereals.
K	Promotes blood clotting.	Green vegetables, vegetable oils, cheese, pork, liver, yogurt.

WHAT MINERALS CAN DO

MINERAL	WHAT IT DOES	WHERE IT CAN BE FOUND
Sodium	A constituent of salt, it helps hold water in the body.	Salt, bread, cereals, bacon, ham.
Potassium	Maintains a normal heart rhythm; helps the function of the nervous system and kidneys.	Fruit, vegetables, meat, milk.
Calcium	Helps blood to clot and keeps bones and teeth healthy.	Milk, green leafy vegetables, beans.
Iron	A constituent of the oxygen-carrying pigment of red blood cells.	Liver, meat, egg yolk, wholegrain cereal, nuts, beans.
Fluoride	Helps harden the teeth and strengthen the bones.	Saltwater fish, tea, coffee, soybeans; added to water in many areas.
Iodine	Aids action of thyroid gland, which controls growth and development.	Saltwater fish, shellfish.

EATING FROM THE FIVE MAIN FOOD GROUPS

To maintain a balanced diet, you need to choose a combination of foods from the five main food groups. The chart below is a guide to the types of food in each group and the nutrients they provide. The chart also includes the recommended guidelines for what you should eat daily and gives tips on how to increase or decrease your intake of particular types of foods.

THE MAIN FOOD GROUPS

FOOD GROUP	WHAT IT CONTAINS	DAILY NEEDS
Cereals and potatoes	Bread, pasta, oats, cereal, potatoes, and rice Good sources of starch and energy; rich in fiber, vitamins, and minerals.	Four portions Boost your intake by eating all types and opt for high-fiber varieties where possible. Try not to eat them with added fat.
Fruit and vegetables	Fruit and vegetables These are a good source of vitamins, minerals, and fiber. Fresh is best, but frozen, dried, and canned can also be eaten.	Four or five portions Eat some fruit and vegetables raw. A glass of fruit juice is one serving. Check canned products for added salt or sugar.
Meat, fish, and alternatives	Fish, nuts, meat, eggs, poultry, tofu, and seeds These foods are good sources of protein, vitamins, and minerals.	Two portions Choose lean cuts of meat, and fish such as salmon and herring. Remove the skin from poultry to reduce the fat content.
Milk and dairy products	Cheese, yogurt, and cream Good sources of calcium and protein, but many products from this group have a high saturated fat content.	Two portions Choose low-fat varieties, such as semiskimmed milk, low-fat yogurt, and cheeses such as Edam.
Fatty and sugary foods	Jam, butter, candy, chocolate, oil, sugar, and chips These are high in calories and provide the body with energy, but many contain saturated fats.	Eat only occasionally This is the only group that should not be eaten on a daily basis. Eat these foods only in small quantities. Try snacking on fruit and vegetables instead.

SPECIAL DIETS

YOU MAY HAVE TO ADAPT your relative's diet for health reasons or to satisfy her personal tastes. Always follow the advice of a nutritionist or physician if your relative's diet is restricted for medical reasons, and respect your relative's wishes if she chooses not to eat certain foods. Whatever types of food you are providing, try to meet the requirements of a balanced diet.

COMBINING PLANT FOODS

Unlike animal foods, no single plant food contains all the amino acids that the body requires. To assist their intake of "complete" proteins, people who do not eat meat need to make sure that they eat plant foods in the correct combinations.

Good combinations

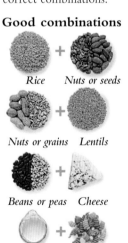

Rice   Nuts or seeds

Nuts or grains   Lentils

Beans or peas   Cheese

Milk   Pasta

Bread   Beans or peas

A DIET FOR HEALTH REASONS

Certain illnesses and conditions can result in dietary restrictions. For example, someone with heart disease may have to reduce salt or fat intake, and a condition such as diabetes may necessitate a controlled sugar intake. A physician or nutritionist will be able to advise on what can and cannot be eaten.

A VEGETARIAN DIET

Vegetarians do not eat meat or fish. Most will eat some animal foods, such as dairy products, but always check the person's preference. A vegetarian diet differs from a nonvegetarian one in several ways.

A low level of saturated fat Because of the absence of red meat in a vegetarian diet, the level of saturated fat will be low.

A high level of fiber The diet is more likely to contain meat alternatives, such as beans, pulses, and grains, and will therefore be high in fiber.

Incomplete proteins There will be a lack of complete proteins because of the absence of meat in the diet (*see left*).

A VEGAN DIET

A person on a vegan diet does not eat meat or dairy products, but uses milk, butter, and cheese made from nuts and soybeans. Like vegetarians, vegans need to combine a range of plant foods to ensure that they are getting sufficient proteins (*see left*). As a result of the absence of certain foods from their diet, they may also need to take vitamin supplements (especially B_{12}). If you are unsure whether or not vitamins are needed, consult a physician or nutritionist.

CULTURAL DIETS

As a volunteer caregiver, you may be looking after someone whose beliefs are different from your own, so it is essential to understand their dietary needs. Fasting may be required on certain days, but in most cultures the infirm, elderly, and babies are excluded from this, especially if the fast involves fluid deprivation. The actual dates for fasting may change from year to year.

SPECIAL CULTURAL REQUIREMENTS		
CULTURE	DIETARY PREFERENCES	RESTRICTIONS
Hindu	◆ Many Hindus are vegetarian. ◆ Beef is never eaten. ◆ Cow's milk is acceptable. ◆ Fasting is common, although fruit, salad without salt, and hot milk or tea are allowed.	◆ May object to utensils that have been used to prepare meat or meat products. ◆ Alcohol and tobacco are forbidden. **Special days in calendar**: Fasting on *Ramanavami* (1 day), *Dushera* (10 days), and *Karva Chauth* (1 day).
Islam	◆ Halal meat (from animals that have been ritually slaughtered according to Muslim law) is eaten. ◆ Muslims do not eat pork or meat from carnivorous animals.	◆ Halal meat should be stored and cooked separately from other products. ◆ Alcohol and tobacco are forbidden. **Special days in calendar**: Fasting during *Ramadan* (30 days) from dawn to dusk, and *Shab-E-Barat* (1 day) three weeks before *Ramadan* begins.
Jewish	◆ Kosher meat (from animals killed and prepared in a certain way) is preferred. ◆ Jews avoid pork, bacon, ham, rabbit, and shellfish. ◆ Meat and poultry must not be served with dairy products.	◆ Separate utensils must be used for dairy and meat products. ◆ Three hours should elapse between eating meat and any dairy product. **Special days in calendar**: Fasting on *Yom Kippur* (25 hours) and food restrictions for Passover (8 days).
Sikhs	◆ Dairy produce is important. ◆ Beef is never eaten. ◆ Many Sikhs are vegetarian, but some can eat meat slaughtered following a rite called *Chakardi*.	◆ Alcohol and tobacco are forbidden. **Special days in calendar**: Some people, often women, fast; they do not avoid all foods, but may reduce the quantity or variety of food eaten for one or two days per week.
Chinese	◆ Believe that health is related to a balance of the body's physical elements (*Taoism*).	◆ Some think that cold food should not be eaten by a sick person or that an illness indicates a need to alter the diet.

MAKING MEALTIMES ENJOYABLE

IDEALLY, A BALANCED DIET is made up of three meals a day but, if this is not possible, you should try to provide the equivalent amount of food and the correct combination of nutrients on a daily basis. To encourage your relative to eat meals, try to provide appetizing food in a relaxed environment and make sure she has the necessary items to enable her to eat without assistance.

PROVIDING FOOD FOR A SICK PERSON

If your relative is sick, she may have little or no appetite. With short-term illnesses, such as a cold or mild flu, eating less is acceptable if sufficient fluid intake is maintained. However, for long-term illnesses, the right amount of food and the correct balance of nutrients is essential to help the body fight disease and repair damage. If you are worried about the level of your relative's food intake, ask her physician if she should have food supplements.

Quantity of food

Three large meals a day may be daunting if your relative does not have an appetite. It is better for her to eat a few small meals than feel defeated because she cannot finish what is on her plate. Give her small portions throughout the day and remove any leftovers immediately. Be patient and encouraging.

PREPARING FOR A MEAL

To maximize her enjoyment, make sure that your relative is comfortable and that everything she needs is within reach. She should have enough room in which to eat her meal – whether she is sitting in a chair, or using a tray or bed table – and the food should look and taste as appetizing as possible.

PROVIDE A RELAXED ENVIRONMENT

Listen to your relative's wishes: she may want music, or the television or radio turned on during her meal. Check whether she would like to use the toilet before eating, and offer her a chance to freshen up. You may want to consider freshening the room with flowers or potpourri. Eating with company can be more enjoyable than eating alone so, if convenient, you or other members of the household should join your relative for a meal.

MAKE SURE THAT MEALS ARE APPETIZING

Where possible, your relative should help decide what will be cooked and, if she is able, encourage her to help prepare the meal.

Think about what you give her Provide foods that she enjoys – and that she is allowed to eat – in small, manageable portions.

Make the food attractive Presentation is important with any meal and can encourage someone who otherwise has little appetite, to eat. Provide a choice of seasonings and relishes, but remember that some items, such as salt, may not be permitted because of a medical condition (*see page 64*). If it does not conflict with dietary restrictions, an alcoholic drink, such as a glass of sherry or wine before or with a meal, may stimulate her appetite.

Adapting for a Physical Impairment

Physical impairment does not necessarily mean that your relative cannot feed herself or enjoy her meals. You can encourage independence by obtaining special aids to suit her specific needs (*see pages 68–69*).

Someone without teeth

If your relative is not able to wear dentures, she will find it difficult to chew, so she will require a diet of soft foods. Prepare foods that can be mashed or use a food processor or blender, if available.

Someone who is bedridden

Make a bedridden person as comfortable as possible, using pillows to help her sit up. Place the items on a bed table or tray (*see page 86*) and check that the bedclothes are properly protected.

Someone who cannot feed herself

If it is necessary to feed your relative, you can help create a more relaxed atmosphere by talking and making her feel more comfortable. If you behave naturally, it will help make both of you feel less self-conscious. When offering the food, make sure you hold the fork or spoon in your relative's line of vision so that she can see what she is eating.

Catering Help

If you are unable to provide meals, perhaps due to illness or because you are away from the house in the daytime, you may be able to get outside help. Seek advice from a care professional to find out what services are available in your area.

Meals on Wheels This service provides a regular midday meal from Monday to Friday (and sometimes at weekends). A financial contribution may be required for each meal.

Day centers If your relative attends a day center, it is likely that she will be provided with a midday meal.

Helping a Visually Impaired Person

Someone who is visually impaired should be able to feed herself, but thoughtful preparation will be required to enable her to be independent. Think about what you prepare – foods such as peas, for example, may be difficult for the person to eat because they slide around the plate.
The "clock" method If you arrange the food on the plate in a certain way, a visually impaired person can have more control over what she is choosing to eat. If she is told where the food is on the plate – for example, the potatoes are at "12 o' clock" – she will be able to eat without your assistance.

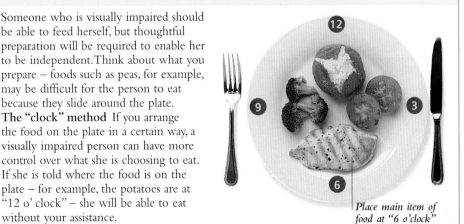

Place main item of food at "6 o'clock"

AIDS TO EATING AND DRINKING

SPECIALIZED AIDS CAN ENABLE SOMEONE who has restricted use of an arm or a hand to prepare food for herself, and to eat and drink without help. These aids range from devices that enable a person to open containers and prepare food, to specially adapted dishes and utensils. The kitchen may also need to be adapted to suit the person's needs (*see page 48*).

PREPARING FOOD

Cutting and spreading aids
Devices that hold food in place are available. For example, bread can be secured while it is spread with butter or sliced. These items are very useful for someone who can use only one hand.
Cooking basket Lifting hot pans can be dangerous for someone who is frail or has a weak grip. By using a cooking basket, the person can lower the food into the hot water and, when it is cooked, simply lift the basket out of the water without having to lift the pan.

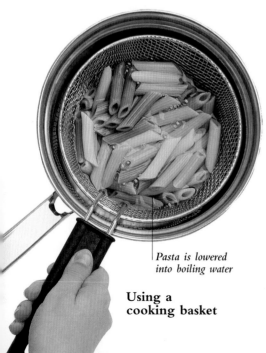

Pasta is lowered into boiling water

Using a cooking basket

OPENING JARS AND BOTTLES

Jar openers A variety of openers with grooves or bands to grip the lids of bottles and jars are available. The openers enable someone with weak hands or wrists to open jars more easily.

Using a grooved jar opener

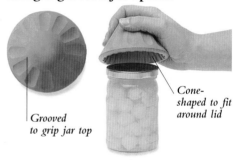

Grooved to grip jar top

Cone-shaped to fit around lid

Using an expandable jar opener

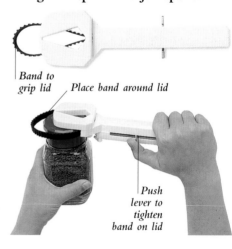

Band to grip lid   *Place band around lid*

Push lever to tighten band on lid

DRINKING AIDS

Cups Drinking from a normal cup can be difficult and dangerous for someone who has a weak grip or is bedridden. Flexible straws and cups with specially designed handles and spouts enable a person to drink safely and without help.

Using a cup with a spout

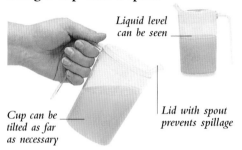

Liquid level can be seen

Cup can be tilted as far as necessary

Lid with spout prevents spillage

Using a hand-rest cup

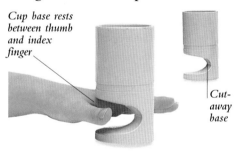

Cup base rests between thumb and index finger

Cut-away base

Using a two-handled cup

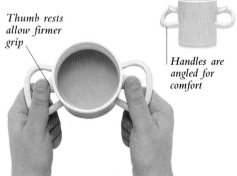

Thumb rests allow firmer grip

Handles are angled for comfort

EATING AIDS

Utensils Specially shaped and thick-handled utensils are designed for someone with a weak grip or someone who only has the use of one hand.

Knife/fork combination

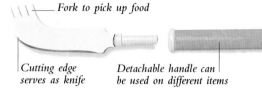

Fork to pick up food

Cutting edge serves as knife

Detachable handle can be used on different items

Spoon/fork combination

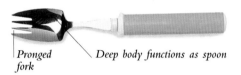

Pronged fork

Deep body functions as spoon

Angled spoon

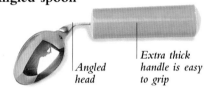

Angled head

Extra thick handle is easy to grip

Plate guard Someone who can use only one hand can get food onto a fork or spoon by pushing it against a plate guard.

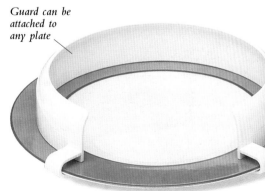

Guard can be attached to any plate

MINOR DIGESTIVE PROBLEMS

IF YOUR RELATIVE IS SICK she may vomit, especially after eating. Steps should be taken to limit any distress this may cause and, if the problem persists, you should seek medical help. An immobile person may have difficulty digesting food, which can lead to a variety of uncomfortable symptoms collectively known as indigestion; as a result her diet and eating habits may need to be changed.

WHY INDIGESTION CAN OCCUR

If your relative's indigestion is due to her inability to chew, provide soft foods and seek the advice of her physician. Indigestion may also be caused by the following:
◆ lying down or bending forward after eating a large meal
◆ eating spicy meals
◆ eating too quickly
◆ either drinking too much alcohol, or drinking alcohol on an empty stomach
◆ smoking

Sites of discomfort

Heartburn is burning sensation in chest

Indigestion is discomfort in upper abdomen

VOMITING

This may be a sign of an underlying infection or illness, so check for other symptoms. If vomiting occurs often, consult your relative's physician, who may ask you for the following information:
◆ the color and content of the vomit (check in particular for any blood)
◆ whether vomiting is linked to eating and drinking
◆ whether there is pain or diarrhea
To help, keep a bowl and washcloth at hand and offer your relative the chance to freshen up afterward.

EATING DISORDERS

Frequent vomiting can indicate eating disorders, such as anorexia nervosa or bulimia. Possible signs are:
◆ regular use of the bathroom after meals
◆ avoiding meals altogether
◆ losing a lot of weight
Seek medical advice if you suspect these disorders.

INDIGESTION AND HEARTBURN

Indigestion usually occurs soon after eating or drinking. The symptoms can vary, but there is often a feeling of fullness and discomfort in the abdomen, perhaps accompanied by burping, nausea, and heartburn. Your relative should take measures to prevent it from occurring.
Pinpoint the cause Try to work out why the indigestion is occurring and avoid the cause.
Neutralize stomach acid The discomfort may be relieved by milk or an over-the-counter antacid (ask a pharmacist to recommend one), but the physician should be consulted if the symptoms persist or recur.

CHAPTER 7

MAINTAINING & IMPROVING MOBILITY

Your relative's ability to walk or move around may be
impeded as the result of an illness or injury, or simply because he
is frail; either way he will be more reliant on you for help.
There are varying degrees of immobility, ranging from difficulty
in getting out of a chair to the inability to stand up or walk. This
chapter demonstrates the correct techniques for helping
your relative move around the home, and illustrates the types of
mobility aids that can encourage independence. An aid, such as
a cane or walker, may enable your relative to undertake routine
activities, such as shopping or visiting friends, by himself. This
level of independence may greatly increase his
confidence and speed up his recovery.

TAKING CARE OF YOURSELF

There are strict guidelines for moving and handling an immobile
person that should be followed closely so that you avoid injuring
yourself. If it is necessary for you to move your relative, make sure
that the correct procedures are demonstrated to you by a
healthcare professional, such as an occupational therapist,
registered nurse, or physical therapist. If your relative is very
immobile, there are special aids and equipment available that are
designed to make it safer and easier for you to move him.

HANDLING SOMEONE SAFELY

IF YOU ATTEMPT TO MOVE YOUR RELATIVE INCORRECTLY, you may hurt yourself – particularly your back – or aggravate your relative's condition. These risks can be avoided if you follow the correct procedures for moving and handling a person. The techniques that are most appropriate for you and your relative should be demonstrated to you by a healthcare professional.

GETTING SPECIALIST HELP

If it is necessary to move your relative regularly, you must get specialist help. If you care for your relative on your own, it is especially important for you to seek advice, since your risk of injury (particularly back strain), or injuring your relative, is increased.

Talking to a professional The physician or nurse practioner can arrange for a specialist, such as a physical therapist or an occupational therapist, to assess your situation and show you the correct procedures for moving your relative.

Using equipment If your relative needs a high level of assistance – for example, if he has to be helped into a bed or a bathtub – you should be shown how to use specialized equipment, such as a hoist (*see page 92*), as well as how to maintain it.

PREPARING TO MOVE SOMEONE

If part of your daily caregiving duties involve moving your relative, always make sure that you are fully prepared for the task. (For guidelines on what you should do if your relative falls down, (*see pages 76–77.*)

The move Is there anyone who can help you?

You Have you been shown how to carry out the move? Are you wearing anything unsuitable – such as high-heeled shoes – that may be dangerous?

Your relative Is your relative mobile enough to help with part of the procedure – is he able to move himself to the edge of a chair, for example?

Safety Do you have enough space to carry out the procedure safely? Are you attempting any procedures that have not been fully explained to you?

SAFETY GUIDELINES

Back strain is one of the most common injuries sustained in the process of moving a person. To prevent this, try to get someone else to help you, and follow these guidelines:

◆ Do not move a person if you have a back injury.

◆ Move him only if it is absolutely necessary.

◆ Reassure the person and tell him what you plan to do.

◆ Explain the task to any helpers and elect one person to give clear instructions.

◆ Employ correct techniques that allow you to use your legs and body weight to provide the power for the move, and thereby avoid straining your back or arms.

◆ Straighten your back when moving the person, and bend your knees, where necessary.

◆ Use equipment or moving and handling aids only if their use has been fully demonstrated to you.

WAYS OF ASSISTING MOBILITY

THE FOLLOWING PAGES SHOW what you can do to help your relative if he has mobility problems. None of the techniques involve *lifting* but, instead, show you how to move your relative by transferring body weight. If a mobility aid has been recommended, encourage him to use it. Procedures for moving your relative in bed are covered in *Bed Comfort* (*see pages 83–96*).

HELPING SOMEONE WALK

Position yourself on the person's weaker side. Support him around the waist with one hand, preferably by grasping his waistband or using a gait belt, and hold the hand closest to you. This position will enable you to support him if he becomes unsteady (*see page 74*).

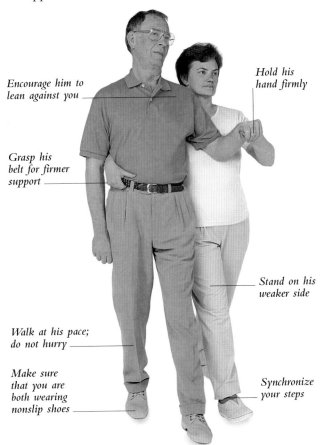

Encourage him to lean against you

Grasp his belt for firmer support

Hold his hand firmly

Walk at his pace; do not hurry

Make sure that you are both wearing nonslip shoes

Stand on his weaker side

Synchronize your steps

CAUSES OF IMMOBILITY

Various conditions can cause immobility. (*See also* Glossary, *pages 178–80*.)

Joint and bone problems Arthritis and rheumatism, and sprained or fractured limbs, will restrict mobility.

Convalescence Those who are weak after an operation or illness may need help to walk.

Conditions of the nervous system This body system controls movement; it is affected by illnesses such as Parkinson's disease and multiple sclerosis.

Heart or breathing complaints Shortness of breath can restrict mobility (*see page 130*).

Stroke One side of the body may be paralyzed because of damage to the brain and nervous system.

Impaired vision Confidence to move around may be affected.

CONTROLLING A FALL

If you are helping your relative walk and you think he is about to fall, you can control his fall using the method below, which involves slow and controlled movements that minimize the risk of injury to you and your relative. Never try to break a fall by catching the person or pulling him over to a chair.

Grasp both of his wrists as he falls

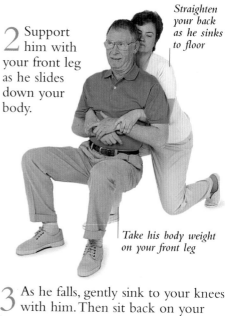

2 Support him with your front leg as he slides down your body.

Straighten your back as he sinks to floor

Take his body weight on your front leg

3 As he falls, gently sink to your knees with him. Then sit back on your heels for better balance, and support his head against your body.

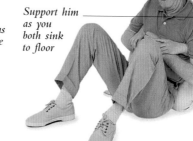

Support him as you both sink to floor

Get behind him as quickly as possible

1 Move behind the person. Grasp his wrists and fold his arms across his chest. With one foot in front of the other, lean into him and allow his weight to fall against your body.

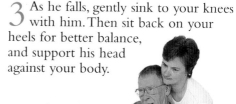

MOVING SOMEONE FROM A WHEELCHAIR INTO A CAR

Open the car door wide and move the passenger seat back. Remove the side of the wheelchair and the footrest nearest the car. Position the wheelchair as close to the car as possible, at a slight angle. Put on the wheelchair brakes. Using the same technique as you would to help someone out of a chair (*see opposite* and *page 78*), stand the person up and pivot him around so that the backs of his legs are against the car. Protect his head from hitting the top of the door frame as you lower him into the car, then gently swing his legs around into the car and make him comfortable.

HELPING SOMEONE OUT OF A CHAIR

If your relative has problems getting up from a chair, it is advisable to invest in a chair with a high seat and firm armrests. The method below can also be carried out using a lifting sling (*see page 78*).

1 Help the person move to the edge of the chair. Stand with your knees on either side of his, and keep your back straight.

Hold onto his belt or waistband

Bend your knees

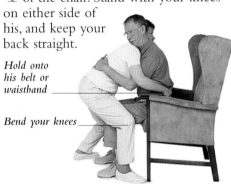

2 Grasp his belt or waistband. Ask him to place his hands around your waist and to rest his head on your shoulder.

3 Begin with a rocking motion and bring your relative up with you on the count of three.

Straighten your back

Straighten your knees

Do not move your feet

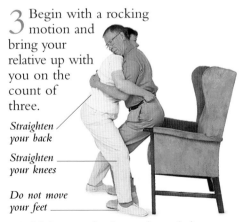

4 Make sure he is steady and that you are both balanced before you release him.

HELPING SOMEONE UP AND DOWN STAIRS

Use the procedures shown below to help your relative up and down stairs. Alternatively, consider installing an extra stair rail or stairlift (*see page 47*).

WALKING UPSTAIRS

Stand two steps below the person. Ask her to hold on to the banister, and keep her steady by putting one hand on each hip. Walk up slowly.

Climb stairs at her pace

WALKING DOWNSTAIRS

Stand two steps below the person, *facing* her. Place your hands on her hips and walk down slowly.

Place your hands on her hips to steady her

For better balance, keep both feet on same step

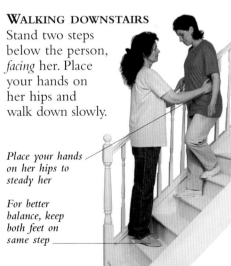

ASSISTING SOMEONE WHO HAS IMPAIRED VISION

Before you offer to guide a visually impaired person, ask her if she would like your help. If you do not know each other, introduce yourself and ask her where she would like to go. **Method** There are two ways to guide the person: either cup your hand under her elbow, or allow her to take your arm; if you are using the latter method, keep your forearm straight and steady. If possible, walk at her side; if not, walk a little ahead, but close enough to maintain contact. Warn her of hazards at head height, and of any changes in ground surface. Tell her when you arrive at the destination and when you are about to leave.

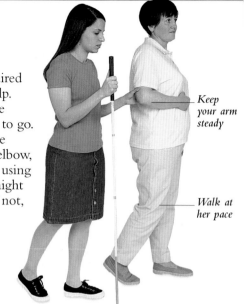

Keep your arm steady

Walk at her pace

HELPING SOMEONE WHO HAS FALLEN

If your relative falls, first deal with any injury and shock (*see pages 147–62*) and, if necessary, call an ambulance. If she is able to move by herself, follow the procedure described opposite to help her back onto her feet. If she is unable to move by herself, do not attempt to move her. If she is in immediate danger – for example, if she has fallen close to water or to a heat source – you may have to move her, but try to get someone to help you.

FOR SOMEONE UNABLE TO MOVE

If your relative falls and is injured, call an ambulance. If she is uninjured but unable to move, do not try to move her on your own. You can use a hoist if you have one (*see page 92*), but only if you have been trained to do so. If not, call an ambulance. Make her comfortable while you are waiting for help.

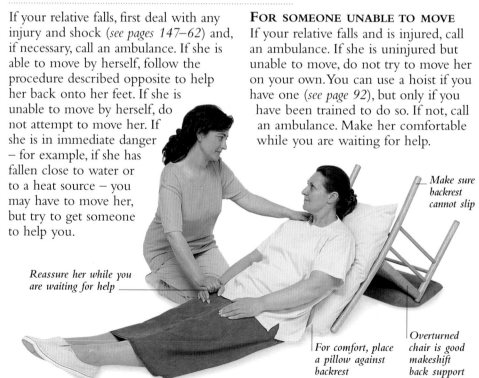

Reassure her while you are waiting for help

Make sure backrest cannot slip

For comfort, place a pillow against backrest

Overturned chair is good makeshift back support

FOR SOMEONE ABLE TO MOVE

If your relative falls but is able to move, you can use the method shown below to help him pull himself into an upright position. This method requires two pieces of sturdy furniture that are different heights – for example, a low stool or a bedside table and an armchair. Place these as close as possible to your relative so that he can support himself and is not in danger of falling again.

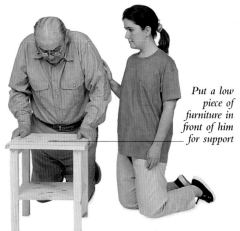

Put a low piece of furniture in front of him for support

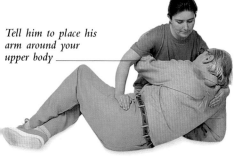

Tell him to place his arm around your upper body

1 Kneel next to the person. Place one hand on his uppermost hip and the other on his shoulderblade. Ask him to grasp you around the upper body.

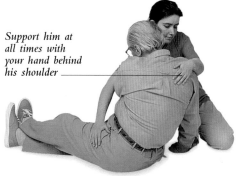

Support him at all times with your hand behind his shoulder

2 Using a rocking motion, on a count of three, press down on his hip and lean back onto your heels. This will assist him to a sitting position.

3 Put a low, sturdy table in front of him and ask him to raise himself to a kneeling position by pushing down on the top of the table. Encourage him to use the table to steady himself.

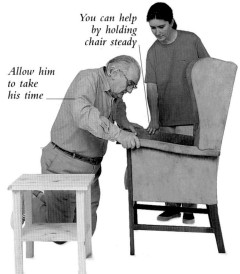

You can help by holding chair steady

Allow him to take his time

4 Place a chair next to the table. Ask him to let go of the table and grasp the arms of the chair. He should now be able to pull himself upright.

MOBILITY AIDS

THERE IS A WIDE VARIETY of equipment available to aid mobility. A healthcare professional, such as a physical therapist, will know what is available and will be able to advise you on the most suitable items for your relative. You may be able to borrow items from a charity organization, local hospital, or hospice, or you may qualify for a loan (*see pages 164–68*).

MOVING AND HANDLING AIDS

The aids shown below make difficult tasks, such as helping someone out of a wheelchair or bed, easier and safer. The products are designed to give you greater control when moving someone, thus minimizing the risk of injury to your back or arms. You should, however, use these items only if you have received proper instruction from a healthcare professional.

Turning disk This is useful for turning your relative around when you help him move from a car into a wheelchair, for example. It works on the principle of one disk rotating over another.

Rubber, nonslip surface prevents person from slipping

To use a turning disk, ask your relative to stand with both feet positioned in the middle of the disk. Rotate him steadily until he is facing the right direction, supporting him all the time.

Walk around with your relative as you rotate him

Lifting aids A lifting strap or sling is used to help someone up from a chair or to sit up in bed. The aid is placed around the person's waist if he is in a chair, or behind his shoulders if he is in bed. (To help someone out of a chair, *see page 75*; to help someone sit up in bed, *see page 88*.)

Lifting strap   **Lifting sling**

Velcro fastening   *Hand grips*

Using a lifting strap

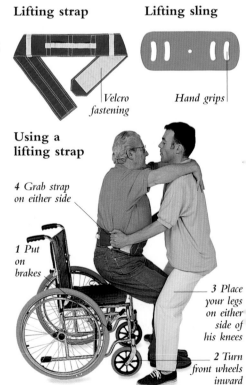

4 Grab strap on either side

1 Put on brakes

3 Place your legs on either side of his knees

2 Turn front wheels inward

WALKING AIDS

The type of aid prescribed will depend on your relative's level of mobility. Canes provide the minimum support, and walkers the maximum. If he has an aid, encourage him to use it whenever possible; this will help him to get used to it and promote independence.

Canes To be the correct height, the curve of the cane should be level with the crease of the wrist when the arm is straight. The person should wear his everyday shoes when it is measured.

Using a cane

If cane is correctly measured, arm should slightly bend to grip it

Crutches These offer stronger support than canes and may be used singly or in pairs. They should be correctly fitted and the person should be shown how to use them.

Using a crutch

Make sure that handgrips are secure

Height can be adjusted

Nonslip rubber tip

Walkers These are available without wheels or with two front wheels. The walker provides firm support, so the user can lean into it and grip it with both hands.

Using a walker

Lightweight aluminum walker

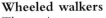

One with wheels is ideal if person cannot lift walker

Wheeled walkers These give support to an unsteady person while allowing him to carry out tasks such as shopping. Some walkers can also be folded flat.

Using a wheeled walker

Hand-operated brake

Basket for shopping

Four wheels make it easy to move

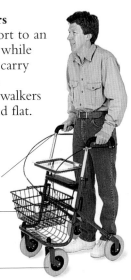

FITTING A WALKING AID

To make sure that walking aids are the correct height for the person using them, they should be measured and fitted by a physical therapist or other trained person. If your relative is having difficulty using an aid, or if it is causing discomfort, seek advice from a healthcare professional.

Wheelchairs

THERE ARE SEVERAL DIFFERENT models of wheelchair available; the type recommended depends on your relative's disability. In most cases, your physician or physical therapist will advise you on the most appropriate type. It may not be necessary to purchase a new wheelchair; you may prefer to rent one instead, or buy a used model.

Choosing a Wheelchair

There are two main types of wheelchair available.
Manual wheelchairs The rider-propelled model has large rear wheels so the user can push himself along; transport chairs have small rear wheels so they need to be pushed. Lightweight folding chairs are also available.
Powered wheelchairs These are used outdoors, indoors, and for long distances.

Wheelchair Safety

To ensure your own safety and the safety of your relative, follow these guidelines:
◆ Never attempt to lift the chair alone with someone in it.

◆ If the chair has a seat belt, make sure it is securely fastened when the chair is in use.

◆ Do not push a wheelchair forward down a step or curb if the person in the chair is at all heavy (*see opposite*).

◆ Check brakes and tire pressures regularly.

◆ Make sure that the user is dressed safely and comfortably (*see page 106*).

Standard self-propelled wheelchair

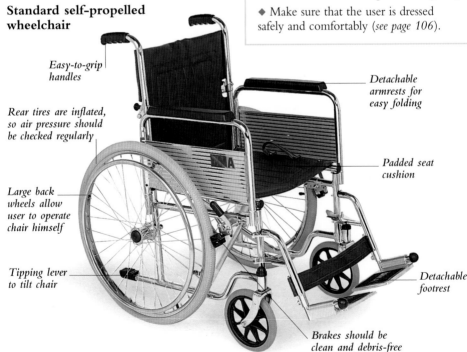

Easy-to-grip handles

Rear tires are inflated, so air pressure should be checked regularly

Large back wheels allow user to operate chair himself

Tipping lever to tilt chair

Detachable armrests for easy folding

Padded seat cushion

Detachable footrest

Brakes should be clean and debris-free

Moving a Wheelchair

When moving a wheelchair up
or down a step or curb, take your
time so that the maneuver is
safe. When tilting the chair, use
the tipping lever.

Going down a step or curb

1 Face the step when
approaching it. Tilt the
wheelchair back by
pushing down on the
tipping lever with
your foot.

2 With the chair tilted,
push the back wheels to
the edge of the curb.

3 Push the chair down the curb
until the back wheels are on the
ground. Then, lower the front wheels
gently onto the ground.

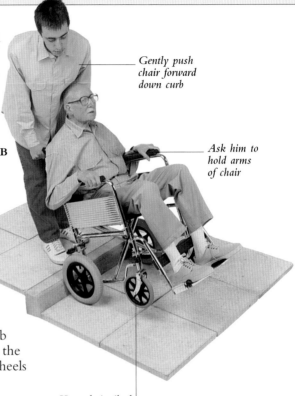

*Gently push
chair forward
down curb*

*Ask him to
hold arms
of chair*

*Keep chair tilted
until back wheels
are on ground*

For a Heavier Person

There is a danger that a heavy occupant
may fall out of the wheelchair if it is
facing forward when you push it down.
You should, therefore, reverse the position
and lower the chair
backward. For this
maneuver, do not
use the tipping
lever to tilt
the chair.

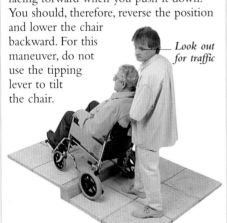

*Look out
for traffic*

Going up a step or curb

1 Face the step or curb when you are
approaching it. Hold the handles of
the wheelchair securely. Place your foot
on the tipping lever in order to tilt the
chair backward.

2 With the wheelchair balanced
on its rear wheels, push it forward
until the front wheels are resting on
the pavement or on the next step up.

3 Use your body weight to push
the wheelchair forward and up the
step until the back wheels are on the
same level as the front. *Never* attempt
to lift the wheelchair.

COMPLICATIONS OF IMMOBILITY

PROLONGED IMMOBILITY may affect your relative's physical or mental health. As a caregiver, you need to be aware of the likely consequences and know how to help prevent or alleviate them. Since debilitating conditions may lead to boredom, anger, depression, and isolation, you will also need to provide emotional support and encourage recreational activities (*see page 124*).

ENCOURAGING MOBILITY

Even if a person has mobility problems, he should be encouraged to undertake some form of exercise to minimize the risk of any complications occurring (*see right*). If your relative is confined to a wheelchair, seek advice from a healthcare professional about exercises designed specifically for wheelchair users.

Encouraging gentle exercise Your relative should be encouraged to:
◆ engage in gentle exercise, such as short walks or swimming in a warm pool; these activities help improve his circulation;

◆ find out about local activities, such as sports or dancing, specifically arranged for people with disabilities;

◆ Begin or continue a hobby, such as gardening, that involves some form of physical activity.

PHYSICAL EFFECTS OF IMMOBILITY

Immobility can lead to other complications, such as infections or poor circulation. It may be possible to minimize these complications by seeking the advice of the physician or nurse practitioner and by following the suggestions below.

Urinary tract infections Sitting for long periods of time may prevent the bladder from emptying properly. Residual urine can stagnate in the bladder, which may result in infection. Encourage your relative to drink plenty of fluids to ensure urine flow.

Constipation Physical inactivity can lead to constipation (*see page 108*), but a high-fiber diet and plenty of fluids can help to minimize this. If the problem persists, seek medical advice.

Chest infections Lying down for long periods causes mucus to stagnate in the lowest part of the chest. Regular changes of position can help to displace the mucus, thereby helping to prevent infection.

Circulatory problems Poor circulation can result from long periods of physical inactivity. Gentle physical therapy may be recommended, or special support stockings may be prescribed. If he complains of any sudden pains in his lower limbs or chest, tell the physician or nurse practitioner immediately.

Pressure sores If your relative's condition results in him lying or sitting in one position for long periods, he is at risk of developing pressure sores (*see page 96*). These occur in areas where skin and tissue are squeezed between the bones and an underlying surface, so blood supply to the tissues is restricted, which starves them of nutrients. To prevent pressure sores, an immobile person should change position (*see page 90*) about every two hours. If pressure sores develop, seek urgent medical treatment.

CHAPTER 8

BED COMFORT

Looking after someone who is confined to
bed can be tiring and time-consuming for you and
frustrating and restrictive for the person affected. This chapter
illustrates several aids and techniques to help you
provide a bedridden person with the safest and
most effective care.

MOVING A PERSON IN BED

You may have to help your relative into and out
of bed, and even change her position once she is in bed. If
you undertake these procedures incorrectly, you may injure both
yourself and your relative. This chapter outlines effective ways of
moving a person in bed; the procedures should, however, be
demonstrated to you by a healthcare professional. If any
specialized equipment is recommended, it is essential that you
be shown how to use it correctly.

REST AND SLEEP

You can improve your relative's quality of life by making
sure that she is as comfortable as possible in bed. This chapter
illustrates bed aids, such as specialized pillows and mattresses, that
are particularly useful for those who have to undergo long periods
of bed rest. It also recommends ways that you can minimize any
physical discomfort or environmental disturbances that may
prevent your relative from getting essential rest and sleep.

BEDS AND BEDDING

LOOK AT WAYS THAT YOUR RELATIVE'S existing bed can be adapted both for her comfort and for your safety and convenience, because purchasing a new one may be disruptive for her. If your relative is in bed for long periods, you will need to change the bedding more often than usual. Make sure that you have enough bedclothes to be able to do this.

SELECTING THE BEST BEDDING

Choose bedclothes that are comfortable, machine-washable, and easy to dry.

Cotton covers Bed-clothes that are 100% cotton or a cotton mix is best because they are less likely to make a person perspire. They can also be washed at high temperatures, which is an important factor if the person has an infectious disease or is incontinent. You will find fitted sheets easier to put on and keep flat.

Blankets Ideally, your relative should have two blankets: a light-weight, cotton or wool blanket for the summer, and a heavier wool blanket for the winter.

Incontinence bedding If you are caring for someone who is incontinent, it is advisable to obtain either a mattress protector or bed protector (*see page 113*).

ADAPTING AND POSITIONING THE BED

To be able to care for someone effectively, the bed needs to be at the right height, not too wide, and positioned so that you can reach both sides easily.
Bed height The mattress should be high enough for you to take care of your relative without having to bend too low. You may wish to use raisers to elevate the bed (*see page 52*), but seek professional advice first.
Bed size It is easier to care for someone in a single bed so that you can reach her easily without over-stretching. If your relative prefers to sleep in a double bed, encourage her to lie on one side of it so that you can reach her more easily.
Position and location Position the bed away from the wall so that you can move around it easily. You may also need to relocate your relative's bedroom if she has difficulty climbing the stairs or so that she can get to the toilet more easily.

MAKING THE BED

When you need to change the sheets, encourage your relative to get out of bed. If she is not able to do this, use one of the methods shown opposite to make the bed. You may want to use a guard rail if available, or position a chair next to the bed, to prevent her from falling off the bed while you are making it.
◆ Remove all the bedding and replace it with clean sheets and pillowcases.
◆ Stretch the bottom sheet to the corners of the bed and smooth away any wrinkles, which could rub against the skin and cause pressure sores (*see page 96*).
◆ Tuck the top sheet in loosely to allow free movement of the feet, which can help prevent pressure sores.
◆ Keep a receptacle nearby for the dirty sheets.

CHANGING SHEETS FOR A BEDRIDDEN PERSON

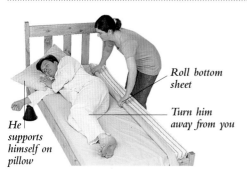

Roll bottom sheet

Turn him away from you

He supports himself on pillow

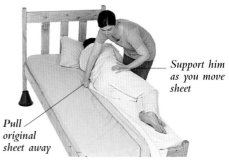

Support him as you move sheet

Pull original sheet away

1 Roll up a clean sheet lengthwise ready to use later. Turn the person onto his side (*see page 90*). Roll the dirty sheet up to his back.

3 Turn the person toward you over the two rolls and onto the clean sheet. Remove the dirty sheet and place it in a laundry bag or hamper.

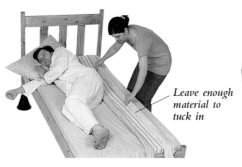

Leave enough material to tuck in

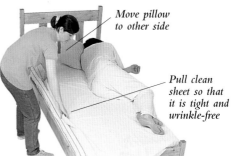

Move pillow to other side

Pull clean sheet so that it is tight and wrinkle-free

2 Place the rolled-up clean sheet on the edge of the bed, open end toward you. Unroll it to where the dirty sheet is placed.

4 Unroll the remainder of the clean sheet across the bed and tuck it in. Then turn him onto his back again and make him comfortable.

FOR SOMEONE WHO CANNOT BE TURNED

If the person cannot lie on his side:
◆ Sit him up and move him down the bed (*see pages 88–89*).
◆ Roll the dirty sheet down to his back.
◆ Replace it with a clean sheet.
◆ Move him back, onto the clean sheet.
◆ Remove the dirty sheet.
◆ Pull the clean sheet from under his legs and tuck it in.

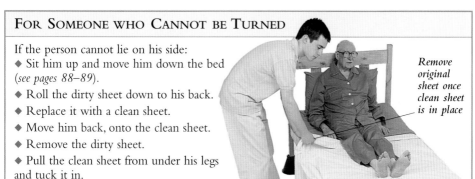

Remove original sheet once clean sheet is in place

AIDS TO COMFORT

IN ADDITION TO SUITABLE BEDDING, you may wish to buy one or two extra items that add to your relative's comfort in bed. Some of these aids prevent pressure sores, while others make activities, such as eating or reading in bed, easier and more enjoyable. An occupational therapist will be able to advise you on the items that are most appropriate for your relative's needs.

BED CRADLES

A bed cradle is placed under the mattress after the bottom sheet is on. The top bedclothes can then be draped over it to keep their weight off the person and prevent pressure sores.

MATTRESSES

Variable-pressure mattresses can be made of spongy material or of a series of air pockets that inflate and deflate independently. Both help to distribute the person's weight evenly so that the points at which the body comes into contact with the mattress are varied, thus helping to prevent pressure sores.

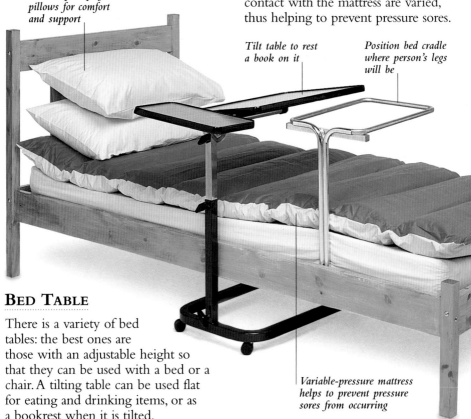

Provide plenty of pillows for comfort and support

Tilt table to rest a book on it

Position bed cradle where person's legs will be

Variable-pressure mattress helps to prevent pressure sores from occurring

BED TABLE

There is a variety of bed tables: the best ones are those with an adjustable height so that they can be used with a bed or a chair. A tilting table can be used flat for eating and drinking items, or as a bookrest when it is tilted.

SUPPORTS

If your relative is confined to bed, it is essential that she sits up for some of the time. This is particularly important to prevent the onset of breathing difficulties and chest infections (*see page 82*). To enable her to sit up, she must have adequate pillow support. Provide plenty of normal pillows, placing them under her head, neck, shoulders, and arms for support, and consider purchasing one of the specialized varieties shown below. For better support, the v-shaped pillow may be needed in conjunction with ordinary pillows.

V-shaped support pillow

This is shaped to provide even support for the neck, back, and arms.

Shaped to support arms

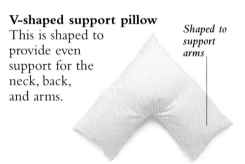

Back support This armchair-shaped support is made from sculptured foam. It enables someone to sit up in bed.

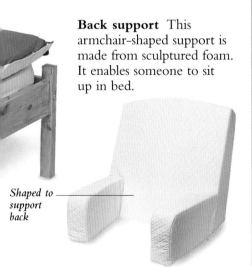

Shaped to support back

HOT-WATER BOTTLE

This provides warmth and comfort, and can help to minimize pain. The bottle should be enclosed in a fleecy cover to prevent it from burning your relative.

Bottle and cover

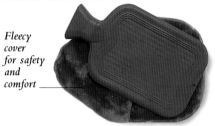

Fleecy cover for safety and comfort

HOW TO FILL A HOT-WATER BOTTLE

Lay the bottle on a flat surface. Holding the neck of the bottle steady, slowly pour in hot, but not boiling, water. Make sure no air pockets form: they can cause hot water to gurgle up and scald you. Fill the bottle ¾ full, gently push out any excess air, and secure the cap. Wipe away any water and put the cover on.

SKIN PROTECTORS

These are made from towels or fleecy fabric. They are designed for people who have to sit in a chair or lie in bed for long periods of time, to wear on areas of the body that are prone to pressure sores, such as the ankles, heels, and elbows.

Ankle and heel protectors

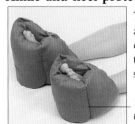

The ankles and heels are cushioned from the hard bed surface.

Velcro makes them easy to fasten

MOVING SOMEONE IN BED

THE TECHNIQUES FOR HELPING your relative into and out of bed, and for changing her position while she is in bed, should be demonstrated to you by a healthcare professional. The methods that you should be shown are outlined here. None of the techniques involve *lifting* but, instead, show you how to move a person by transferring body weight.

> ### SAFETY GUIDELINES
>
> Even if your relative is not heavy, *never* attempt to *lift* her from or in the bed because this may injure your back and arms. If you have not been shown the correct techniques for moving her, find someone to show you. Do not move anyone by yourself if you can get help. Before beginning a move, always explain to your relative what you intend to do.

HELPING SOMEONE TO SIT UP IN BED

1 Face the person. Place one knee on the bed, level with her waist. Fold her arms across her chest. Slide a lifting sling (*see page 78*) under her shoulders. If you do not have one, use your hands instead.

Grasp handles of lifting sling

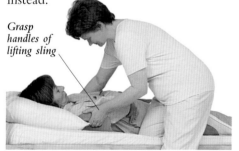

2 Using a rocking motion, lean back onto your heel on the count of three; this will transfer the person's body weight to you, bringing her upright.

Straighten your back

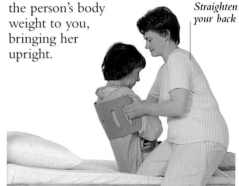

SITTING SOMEONE UP WITH HELP

Position yourself on the bed as shown above and ask your helper to do the same on the other side. Ask the person to fold her arms across her chest. Place one hand under her forearm and the other hand on her shoulder blade; ask your helper to do the same on the other side. Working together, use a rocking motion and lean back on your heels on the count of three to bring the person to a sitting position.

Place one hand on shoulder blade

Place other hand on arm

Her legs should be straight

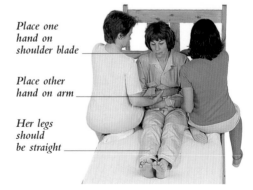

MOVING SOMEONE UP A BED ON YOUR OWN

You may need to move your relative up or down the bed so that you can change the sheets, for example (*see page 85*). The technique shown below allows you to use your body weight to power the move, so that you don't strain your arms and back. However, the technique is only effective if your relative is able to assist by pushing down on the bed with her feet.

1 Help the person sit up (*see opposite*). Ask her to raise her knees.

2 Facing the same direction as she is, place the knee closer to her about 2in (5cm) behind her buttocks.

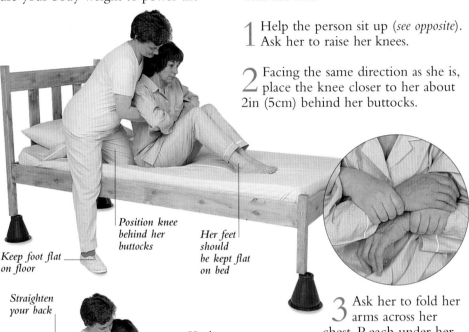

Position knee behind her buttocks

Her feet should be kept flat on bed

Keep foot flat on floor

Straighten your back

Her legs straighten as you move back

Move your leg back

Keep foot in same position

Bed risers elevate bed, thereby making move easier

3 Ask her to fold her arms across her chest. Reach under her arms and grasp her wrists gently, but firmly.

4 Ask her to get ready to push her feet down on the bed on the count of three. Keep your foot on the ground stationary and lean back onto the heel of your bent leg, to transfer her weight and bring her up the bed.

CHANGING SOMEONE'S

POSITION IN BED

If your relative is confined to bed for long periods and cannot move herself, you will need to change her position approximately every two hours to prevent pressure sores from developing. The procedure below shows you how to move your relative, with the aid of a helper, so that she can be turned on her side. Alternatively, you can obtain a sliding sheet (*see page 92*) that will enable you to move her by yourself.

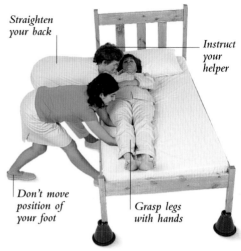

Straighten your back

Instruct your helper

Don't move position of your foot

Grasp legs with hands

1 Slide your hands, palms downward, under the natural hollows of the person's upper body – the shoulders and small of the back. Ask your helper to slide her hands under the lower hollows – the thighs and knees.

3 On a count of three, both straighten your front legs and transfer your weight onto your back legs; the person will move across as you lean back.

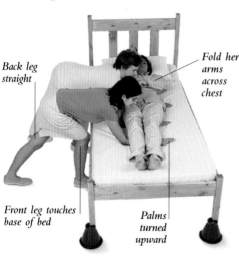

Back leg straight

Fold her arms across chest

Front leg touches base of bed

Palms turned upward

2 Position yourself with one leg in front of the other, with your back leg straight and your front leg bent and touching the base of the bed. Turn your palms upward. Ask your helper to mirror your leg position.

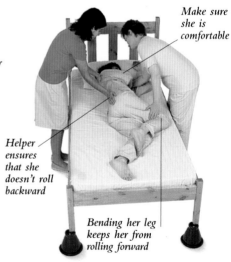

Make sure she is comfortable

Helper ensures that she doesn't roll backward

Bending her leg keeps her from rolling forward

4 Grasp the person's far leg and shoulder to turn her onto her side. Ask your helper to support her from behind as she is turned. Then, support her back and top leg with pillows, if needed. Cover her with bedding.

HELPING SOMEONE GET OUT OF BED

Encourage your relative to get out of bed as often as possible, even if it is only to sit in a chair; it may be detrimental to her health to stay in bed for long periods. The method below can also be used if you want to move her to the edge of the bed to change her nightwear.

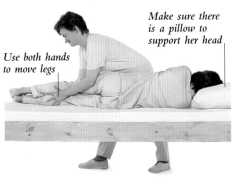

Use both hands to move legs

Make sure there is a pillow to support her head

1 Turn the person onto her side (*see opposite*). Stand beside the bed, level with her waist. Place your hands behind her knees and gently draw her legs out of the bed so that they dangle down toward the floor.

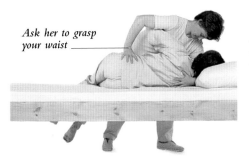

Ask her to grasp your waist

2 Ask her to place her upper arm around your waist; do not let her grasp you around your neck. Place one of your hands on her hip and the other hand on her shoulder blade.

MOVING FROM A BED

Once you have positioned your relative on the side of her bed, you may want to move her to a chair, wheelchair, or commode, or just help her stand up. There are various ways you can do this, but, ideally, you should seek the advice of a healthcare professional, who should be able to advise you on equipment and the best technique for your relative's needs.

Helping her into a standing position Using the technique for getting someone out of a chair (*see page 75*), raise your relative to a standing position. Alternatively, to make the task easier, you could use a device such as a lifting sling (*see page 78*).

Helping her into a chair Once your relative is standing, help her to turn around and sit in the chair (or wheelchair or commode). Alternatively, use a turning disk (*see page 78*). The person stands on this and is gently swiveled around so that she is facing in the correct direction to be seated.

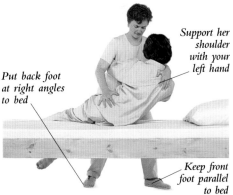

Put back foot at right angles to bed

Support her shoulder with your left hand

Keep front foot parallel to bed

3 Press down on her hip and lean back onto your back leg as you do this. This movement will bring the person to a sitting position. Make sure she is steady before you let go of her.

MOVING AND HANDLING AIDS

THERE IS A VARIETY OF AIDS that can be used to help a person who has restricted mobility in bed: some are designed to make the caregiver's task safer and easier, while others enable an immobile person to be more independent. You may be able to rent or borrow bed aids from a local medical supplier or charity, which can be ideal if they are only needed for a short time.

AIDS THAT HELP A CAREGIVER MOVE SOMEONE

If your relative needs regular help to get into and out of bed, or you have to change her position in bed, you will probably be advised by an occupational therapist to obtain equipment to help move her. The way in which the equipment is operated and installed can vary, depending on the type used, especially for a device such as a hoist. Always ask for a demonstration and read the manufacturer's instructions before attempting to use any device.

Sliding sheet This is a piece of material, with a slippery surface, that allows you to move a person across the bed when she needs to be turned (*see page 90*). You slide it underneath her and, as you pull it toward you, she is automatically moved across with it.

Hoist This is an essential piece of equipment if your relative has to be moved regularly from a chair to a bed, or into a bathtub, for example. Most hoists involve sitting the person in a sling and, once she is securely in place, operating a winch system to lift her. A healthcare professional can advise you on the hoist that is most suitable, and demonstrate how it should be used.

She is slowly moved into position

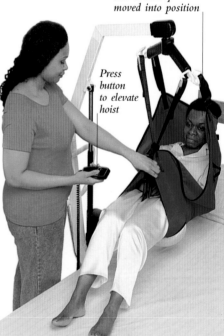

Press button to elevate hoist

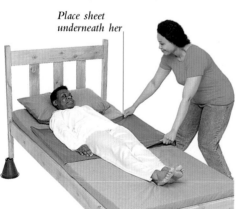

Place sheet underneath her

DEVICES THAT SOMEONE CAN USE UNAIDED

The aids shown here will help a person with some upper body strength to sit up and move around the bed without help.

Bed blocks These are "blocks" with handles that enable a person to move up and down a bed herself, or raise herself, onto a bedpan, for example. You can improvise bed blocks by tying two or three similar-sized books together.

Trapeze bar This is another device that is used to help a person with limited strength to sit up, adjust her position, and get into and out of bed. It is suspended from a strong frame that sits under the head of a bed.

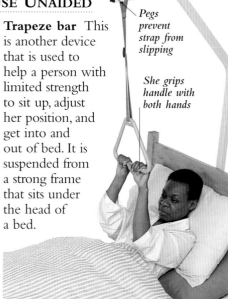

Pegs prevent strap from slipping

She grips handle with both hands

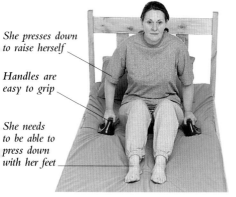

She presses down to raise herself

Handles are easy to grip

She needs to be able to press down with her feet

Rope ladder This device enables a person with reasonably strong hands and arms to raise himself to a sitting position. One end of the ladder is fastened to the bottom end of the bed; the user then pulls on the rungs.

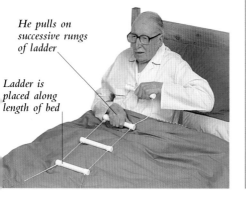

He pulls on successive rungs of ladder

Ladder is placed along length of bed

ADJUSTABLE BEDS

There are various mechanical beds that can be hand-operated to enable a person who has limited mobility to sit up, change position, and get out of bed without help. Some types are fitted with a hand pump, others with an electric motor, enabling the person to adjust the head, back, knee, and foot sections of the bed to the most suitable position.

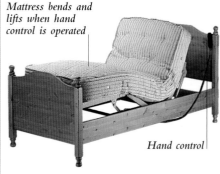

Mattress bends and lifts when hand control is operated

Hand control

Rest and Sleep

IT IS ESSENTIAL FOR YOUR RELATIVE to get enough rest and sleep to restore energy, help the recovery process, and improve morale. Get to know her sleep patterns and, in times of wakefulness or restlessness, try to determine whether the cause is due to physical discomfort, anxiety, or environmental disturbances. Sleeping pills should be taken only if prescribed by a doctor.

Physical and Psychological Discomfort

If your relative cannot get comfortable or relax, she may have difficulty sleeping. It is important that her bed is comfortable, that any pain or physical discomfort is minimized and that she is not kept awake by anxiety. Make sure she has everything she needs within reach, such as nighttime medication and a drink; this may help minimize the length of time that she stays awake. She may also want a book so that she can read herself to sleep.

Solving Physical and Emotional Problems

Problem	Why it Occurs	Solutions
Hunger or thirst	If a person wakes up in the middle of the night, hunger and thirst can prevent her from getting back to sleep.	Make sure she has enough to eat and drink during the day. Place a drink and snack on her bedside table at night.
Physical discomfort	The bed or bedding itself may be uncomfortable and aggravate physical problems. Wakefulness may also be caused by physical discomfort, such as aching limbs, stiff joints, or a full bladder.	Make your relative comfortable in bed. Check that bedding is not too heavy, sheets are not wrinkled or wet, and pillows are a comfortable height. An immobile person should be provided with a toilet aid, such as a commode (*see page 114*).
Pain	Pain in the middle of the night may cause psychological as well as physical discomfort.	Make sure she has taken the correct dosage of pain-relief medicine and that any painkillers required are within her reach.
Anxiety	A person may be kept awake because she is depressed or worried about her illness or a forthcoming operation.	Encourage your relative to talk about her concerns. Find ways for her to relax before bedtime, such as by listening to music or reading a book or magazine.

ENVIRONMENTAL DISTURBANCES

A change of environment may make your relative feel very disorientated, which can disrupt her sleep patterns. To minimize this, try to keep her bedtime routine as familiar as possible. If you have very noisy neighbors, explain to them that your relative needs to rest; you will find that most people will be sympathetic. You might also purchase earplugs for your relative – they are available from pharmacies – especially if she likes to sleep during the day or goes to bed early.

SLEEP PATTERNS

Your relative should not become overtired because it may hinder her recovery. Try to keep to her natural pattern of sleeping, and encourage her to follow this as closely as possible. If she is prevented from taking a customary nap in the afternoon, for example, she may want to sleep in the evening, which may then make it difficult for her to sleep during the night. Make sure that you are not deprived of sleep as well. If you get very tired, try to adapt your own sleep patterns around those of your relative: when she sleeps, use the opportunity to sleep or rest yourself.

MINIMIZING ENVIRONMENTAL DISTURBANCES

PROBLEM	WHY IT OCCURS	SOLUTIONS
Light	The room is too light or too dark at night.	If it is too dark, open the curtains or leave a light on. If it is too light, put up thicker curtains or line existing ones.
Odors	If the room has a strong smell, it can disturb sleep.	Leave a window or door ajar so air can circulate. Use potpourri or flowers to freshen the room.
Change of environment	Your relative is not in her usual room, or has been relocated to a different building altogether.	If your relative is staying elsewhere, ensure that the rest of her bedtime routine remains as undisturbed as possible to minimize the disruption.
Room temperature	Your relative is too hot or too cold at night.	Open or close windows and adjust heating and bedding as necessary; check her body temperature (*see page 128*).
Noise	Noises outside and inside the house can disturb normal sleep patterns.	Try to remove the source of the noise; "soundproof" the room by stuffing a rolled-up sheet or towel along the gap under the door; or provide earplugs.

PRESSURE SORES

WHEN SOMEONE HAS TO SPEND long periods of time in a bed or chair, she may be vulnerable to developing pressure sores. These sores occur in areas where the skin and underlying tissue are compressed between a surface and the bone, cutting off the blood supply to the affected area. Taking simple precautions can minimize the likelihood that pressure sores will develop.

PREVENTING PRESSURE SORES

The following steps can help prevent sores from developing:

◆ Encourage the person to get out of bed as much as possible.

◆ Encourage her to move regularly. If she has very limited mobility, you will need to change her position every two hours (*see page 90*).

◆ Always move the person in the proper way (*see pages 88–89*); do not drag her limbs up or down the bed.

◆ Never allow her to lie or sit in wet or damp conditions.

◆ Make sure the bedding is not irritating her skin and wash the bedclothes regularly.

◆ Ensure that she is eating a balanced diet (*see page 61*).

◆ Inform the physician or registered nurse about any skin changes, such as redness, dryness, or cracking.

VULNERABLE AREAS

If your relative is weak or unconscious, and therefore unable to move in bed, there is a risk that pressure sores might develop. These occur in places where the bones are very near the surface of the skin. The weight of the body reduces the blood supply to the skin tissues, causing the skin to change color, initially to a pinky red. Areas that are vulnerable include:

◆ the head
◆ the shoulders
◆ the elbows
◆ the base of the spine
◆ the hips
◆ the heels and ankles

CAUSES OF PRESSURE SORES

Your relative may be vulnerable to pressures sores if:

◆ she remains in one position for too long;
◆ she has lost a lot of weight through illness, and therefore has less body fat to cushion the bones;
◆ there is friction on the skin, caused by the top sheet being too tight or by her being dragged across the bed, especially if her skin is not clean and dry.

WHAT ACTION YOU SHOULD TAKE

Pressure sores require swift medical attention. If you notice an area that is red, or one that appears blistered and tender, for over 24 hours, inform a healthcare professional, who will determine whether treatment is required. If the skin has broken, the sore is more prone to infection and may take longer to heal. In addition to treating the sores, the physician or registered nurse may suggest that you use pressure-relieving aids (*see pages 86–87*).

CHAPTER 9

PERSONAL CARE

It is essential to your relative's self-esteem and
self-respect that she be able to stay clean and dress herself. This
will help her feel better about herself and to cope more
positively with her condition.

ENCOURAGING INDEPENDENCE

Your support and encouragement are essential,
especially if she is relearning basic skills that she once took for
granted, such as brushing her teeth or putting on socks and shoes.
Encourage her to carry out as many of the tasks as she can on
her own and resist the urge to help, even if she is taking
a long time. She may benefit from using some of the aids shown
in this chapter; an occupational therapist will be able to advise you
on which items are most suitable.

HELPING YOUR RELATIVE

It may be necessary for you to help your relative
wash and dress. In this situation you need to find the safest and
easiest ways to do this and, if necessary, seek advice from
a healthcare professional, such as a nurse practitioner or an
occupational therapist. If your relative is confined to
bed, you may be shown how to give a bedbath; if she has
severe mobility problems and you do not have a showerstall, an
occupational therapist may recommend the use of certain
equipment to help you move her into and out of the bathtub.

HELPING SOMEONE TO WASH

ALWAYS ENCOURAGE YOUR RELATIVE to, at the very least, wash her hands and face at a sink by herself. If she has mobility problems or is weak, you may have to adapt the bathroom to enable her to use it by herself (*see page 50*). If it is necessary to help her into a bathtub, always seek advice about the safest way to do this; an adapted showerstall may be a safer option.

HELPING SOMEONE TO HAVE A SHOWER

An immobile person who cannot climb into a bathtub should be encouraged to use a showerstall. If she has difficulty standing in the shower, obtain a shower seat (*see page 51*); if she is confined to a wheelchair, a chair can be obtained that can be wheeled into and out of the showerstall. It is also advisable to fit handrails and obtain a nonslip mat for the floor.

You can help your relative by:
♦ ensuring that she has all her toiletries;
♦ turning on the water and making sure it is the correct temperature;
♦ passing her the shower head once she is securely seated.
Leave her alone unless she needs assistance and supervision throughout. Agree beforehand on a way for her to communicate that she has finished.

HELPING SOMEONE TO HAVE A BATH

If your relative cannot climb into the bathtub by herself, you may have to help her. Do not, however, attempt to lift her into or out of the tub. Seek the advice of a healthcare professional, who may suggest the use of specialized equipment, such as a hoist (*see page 92*) or bath lift, to enable you to move her. If your relative's mobility is only slightly impaired – she is just generally weak, for example – she may benefit from the use of some simple aids.

Grab rails The person can hold onto these as she gets into and out of the tub.
Nonslip mat This is placed in the bottom of the bathtub to prevent the person from slipping as she gets in and out, and while she is sitting in the tub.
Bath board This is placed across the bathtub so that the person does not have to turn or stretch to reach items.
Bath seat This is placed in the tub so that the person does not have to lower or raise herself as far.

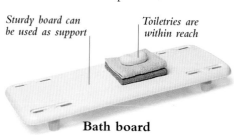

Sturdy board can be used as support *Toiletries are within reach*

Bath board

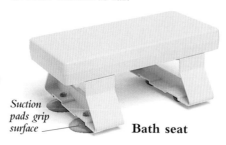

Suction pads grip surface **Bath seat**

GIVING SOMEONE A BEDBATH

Your relative will require a bedbath if he is unable to get out of bed to wash. You will need a bowl of warm water, two or three towels, soap, and two sponges or washclothes; use different sponges for the face and genitals. Keep him warm by covering those parts of the body that are not being washed with a sheet and towel.

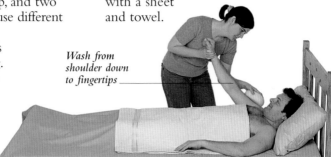

1 Remove the person's upper-body clothing. Pull the top sheet up to his armpits and cover it with a towel. Wash his face, neck, shoulders, arms, and hands, and then dry these areas.

Wash from shoulder down to fingertips

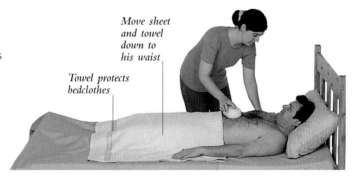

2 Fold the sheet and towel down to his waist. Wash and dry his chest and abdomen; make sure that you dry thoroughly under any folds of skin since sores may develop in areas that remain damp or wet.

Move sheet and towel down to his waist

Towel protects bedclothes

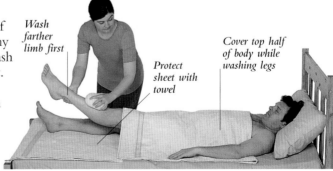

3 Cover the top half of his body. Remove any lower-body clothing. Wash and dry his legs and feet. Allow him to wash the genital area himself with the second sponge. Cover him with the sheet, while you change the water.

Wash farther limb first

Protect sheet with towel

Cover top half of body while washing legs

4 Turn the person onto his side (*see page 90*). Use the original sponge to wash his back and buttocks. Dry him and help him dress in clean clothes.

IF someone has difficulty lying on his side, sit him up (*see page 88*). Protect the bottom sheet with a towel and then wash and dry his back.

WASHING AIDS

STIFF JOINTS, POOR BALANCE, or a general lack of mobility may make it
difficult for your relative to wash herself. To enable her to clean all parts
of her body thoroughly, you can purchase specialized washing aids: the most
useful features are long handles to minimize the amount of stretching required,
and straps for those who have difficulty gripping objects.

USEFUL ITEMS FOR WASHING

Specially adapted washing aids are
useful for those who have difficulty
bending or stretching, and for those
who cannot grip a normal sponge,
brush, or washcloth. Several items are
shown below. Most of these items can
be obtained from a pharmacy; if what

you need is not in stock, it may be
possible to order it. Choose items that
are easy to clean. If you are not sure
which aids are the most suitable for the
person in your care, ask an occupational
therapist, who is trained to determine
individual requirements.

Washcloth strap

_Strap allows a person to
keep her hand flat_

This item is useful for a person who
cannot grip a washcloth. She holds it
by pushing her fingers under the strap.

Long-handled brush

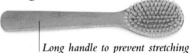

Long handle to prevent stretching

Sweeping along the arms and legs with
this soft-bristled brush can slough dead
skin and stimulate circulation.

Long-handled sponge

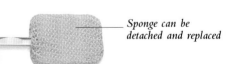

_Sponge can be
detached and replaced_

This soft sponge attached to a long
handle is designed to reach awkward
areas such as the legs, feet, and back.

Length of handle can be adjusted

Back strap

A long strap of padded washcloth enables a
person with limited mobility to wash parts
of the body she finds difficult to reach.

_Padded washcloth is
soft on skin_   _Hoop handles
                       are easy to grip_

CARE OF GENERAL APPEARANCE

I N ADDITION TO STAYING CLEAN, it may be important to your relative's self-esteem to look as presentable as possible – even if she is feeling sick. Using makeup does not have to be part of her daily routine if she does not want it to be, but when people are visiting, or when she is going out shopping or to the day center, it may help to boost her confidence.

APPLYING MAKEUP

You can obtain several useful items that can help your relative to apply makeup without your help.

Magnifying mirror A closer and clearer view can be achieved with a magnifying mirror propped up on a stand for easy use.

Foam tubing Specialized tubing can be attached to items such as lipsticks, eye pencils, and mascaras, to make them easier to grip and thereby easier to apply.

Makeup bag Attach a long ring pull to the zipper on a makeup bag, or replace the zipper with velcro, so that someone who has difficulty gripping can open and close it easily.

Containers It may be better to purchase creams and lotions in jars because a person with limited dexterity may find it difficult to squeeze a tube.

HELPING SOMEONE TO SHAVE

If you are caring for a man, you may need to help him shave. Always ask him whether he would prefer a wet shave or an electric shave. An electric razor may be easier for you to use if you are not experienced or confident in the art of giving a wet shave. Always make sure that the equipment is clean.

GIVING A WET SHAVE

You will need a razor, shaving cream or soap, and water. Rub the soap or foam into a lather over the area to be shaved. Then, holding the skin taut with one hand, firmly pull the razor down the cheek in long strokes, in the direction in which the hair grows. The razor should be sharp enough to cut the stubble, not scrub across his face. Rinse the razor after every few strokes. Rinse the face when you have finished.

USING AN ELECTRIC RAZOR

The hand-over-hand method gives some independence to a person who is able to grip an electric razor, but unable to rotate it. Once he is holding the razor, place your hand over his to direct it.

Using the hand-over-hand method

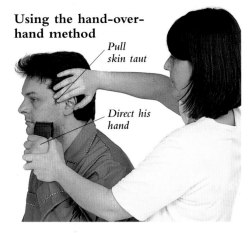

Pull skin taut

Direct his hand

CARING FOR THE HAIR

C LEAN AND GROOMED HAIR, even if it is just simply brushed to remove snarls and styled so that it is neat and manageable, may have a significant effect on how your relative feels about herself. A shampoo, especially, can be very refreshing and uplifting. Regular haircuts will make hair easier to manage – if your relative is housebound, find a hairdresser who can come to your home.

GENERAL HAIR CARE

Unless your relative is very weak, she should be encouraged to brush or comb her hair by herself.

Brushing hair If your relative's condition requires her to lie or sit in the same position for long periods of time, her hair may become tangled. Lying on tangled hair may cause the scalp to become sore, possibly resulting in pressure sores (*see page 96*). To prevent

this from occurring, encourage your relative to brush or comb her hair gently, at least twice a day.

Wig care Your relative may have had treatment that has led to hair loss, such as chemotherapy (*see page 123*). If she wishes to wear a wig, consult a specialist for advice. Wash artificial wigs by hand; natural hair wigs should be washed and styled by a hairdresser.

WASHING HAIR

Having her hair washed can be very refreshing for someone who is sick. Your relative should wash her hair in the bath or shower, if possible. Ask the pharmacist for a dry shampoo or no-rinse shampoo so she can keep her hair clean between washes.

For someone confined to bed If your relative cannot get up, you can obtain a device to wash her hair while she is lying in bed (*see right*). Alternatively, you can wash it by:
♦ laying plastic sheeting or towels over the bed and floor;
♦ positioning the person so that she is sitting up and leaning over a bowl on a bed table. If it is difficult for her to sit up, she can lie with her head over the bottom end of the bed, pillows under her neck and shoulders, and a bowl beneath her head.

HAIR WASHING TRAY

This inflatable tray allows a person to lie flat while his hair is being washed; it is especially useful for someone who has very limited mobility. Place a bowl under the hose to collect the water that drains from the tray.

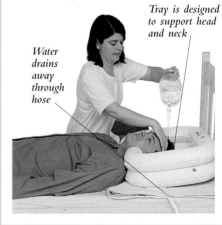

Tray is designed to support head and neck

Water drains away through hose

GENERAL BODY CARE

MEDICATION, SOME COURSES OF TREATMENT, and general immobility may lead to uncomfortable physical side effects. Many of the more common complaints, such as mouth ulcers and eye infections, are treatable at home, as the chart below indicates. There may also be steps you can take to keep the side effects from occurring in the first place. Always seek medical advice, if necessary.

TREATING AND PREVENTING COMMON COMPLAINTS

AREA	COMMON COMPLAINTS	RECOMMENDED CARE
Mouth	◆ Cheek and gum ulcers caused by poor-fitting dentures. ◆ Lack of or excessive salivation, possibly as the result of a stroke. ◆ Poor oral hygiene, cold sores, dehydration, and dry tongue.	◆ Consult a dentist about getting new dentures for your relative. ◆ Provide plenty of fluids and fresh fruit to encourage salivation. ◆ Encourage your relative to brush her teeth thoroughly and provide mouthwashes.
Eyes	◆ Difficulty blinking or closing the eyes as a result of a stroke. ◆ Eye infection.	◆ Wash around the eyes carefully. ◆ Drops or ointments may be prescribed to treat infection (*see page 135*).
Nose	◆ Blocked nose and sore nostrils from cold symptoms.	◆ Drops may be prescribed to relieve congestion (*see page 135*), or creams to soothe soreness.
Feet	◆ Corns, bunions, and blisters. ◆ Fungal infections, such as athlete's foot. ◆ Pressure sores.	◆ Consult a physician for fungal infections; otherwise, consult a podiatrist. ◆ Take steps to prevent pressure sores (*see page 96*) and seek medical advice.
Nails	◆ Hard, brittle nails, prone to splitting, on fingers and toes. ◆ Ingrowing toenails.	◆ Seek the advice of a podiatrist. ◆ Trim nails regularly, cutting straight across and not down into the corners.
Ears	◆ Excessive wax, which may be soft or hard. ◆ Sores on the edge of the ears.	◆ Drops may be prescribed (*see page 135*). ◆ Take steps to prevent pressure sores (*see page 96*) and seek medical advice.
Skin	◆ Red, sore skin in the armpits, groin, or breast areas. ◆ Dry, flaky skin. ◆ Rash caused by allergy.	◆ Ensure that skin in these areas is kept dry. Do not allow talcum powder to clog. ◆ Moisturize regularly. ◆ Seek medical advice – an emollient cream may be prescribed.

DRESSING TECHNIQUES

IF YOUR RELATIVE'S MOBILITY OR DEXTERITY is impaired, the simple tasks of dressing and undressing may be frustrating and exhausting. Losing the ability to dress oneself – to put on a shirt or pull on a sock – can deal a severe blow to a person's independence and dignity. Dressing aids are designed to enable a weak or immobile person to dress herself more easily.

DRESSING AIDS

Most dressing gadgets are designed with long handles to prevent someone with limited mobility from having to bend when she is dressing or undressing herself, thereby minimizing the risk of injuries sustained by falling or over-stretching. All the items shown here are inexpensive and easy to use. An occupational therapist will be able to advise you on the products that are most suited to your relative's needs.

Dressing stick The double wire hook at one end enables a person to pull on or push off clothing. This aid is useful for someone with weak limbs.

Long-handled shoe horn This enables a person to put on her shoes without having to bend, thus minimizing any risk of strain.

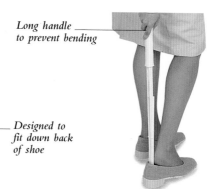

Long handle to prevent bending

— Designed to fit down back of shoe

Stocking aid The stocking is placed over the shaped plastic and then pulled up by pulling the straps.

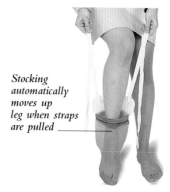

Stocking automatically moves up leg when straps are pulled

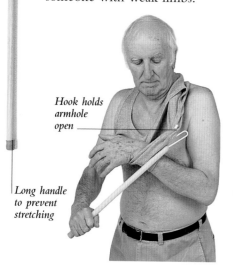

Hook holds armhole open

Long handle to prevent stretching

HELPING SOMEONE TO DRESS

Dressing and undressing can be a lengthy process for a weak or paralyzed person. If possible, allow your relative to dress independently, but if he needs help, follow these guidelines:
◆ make sure he is sitting or lying down to make the task easier;
◆ dress the weak limb first;
◆ always place a garment over the arm before pulling it over the head;
◆ allow him to assist, if at all possible, but do not rush him.

HELPING TO PUT ON SOCKS

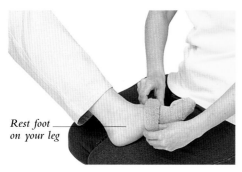

Rest foot on your leg

1 Fold over the top of the sock. Roll it back to halfway along the foot section and place it over the toes.

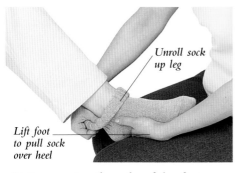

Unroll sock up leg

Lift foot to pull sock over heel

2 Supporting the sole of the foot, unroll the sock over the foot, heel, and up the leg.

DRESSING A PERSON WHO HAS AN INJURED ARM

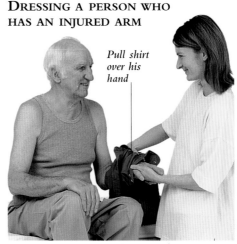

Pull shirt over his hand

1 Roll the sleeve down to the cuff. Place your hand through the cuff opening and grasp the person's hand. Pull the shirt from your own hand over his.

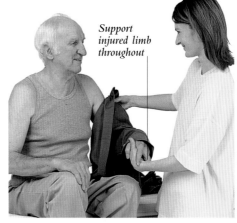

Support injured limb throughout

2 Keep hold of his hand and gently pull the shirt sleeve up his arm to the shoulder.

3 Take the garment around his back, so that he can reach the other sleeve with his good arm. He can then continue dressing by himself.

CHOOSING CLOTHES

IDEALLY, LET YOUR RELATIVE CHOOSE the clothes she would like to wear; if she relies on you to buy them for her, always opt for colors and fabrics that you know she likes. In addition to buying items that are comfortable, consider what is practical: for example, if your relative has dexterity problems, do not buy garments with small buttons or back pockets.

FEATURES TO LOOK FOR

Choose items that may enable a person to dress without help. For example:
◆ slip-on shoes
◆ v-necked sweater
◆ sweatshirt or T-shirt
◆ wraparound skirt
◆ clip-on tie
If your relative has dexterity problems or is weak, consider how difficult she may find it to manipulate the fastenings on garments (*see right*).

FOR WHEELCHAIR USERS

People who are wheelchair bound often find that their waist and hips broaden; users of manual chairs find that their shoulder and upper arm muscles also get bigger. It may, therefore, be necessary for them to wear larger clothing. For safety and comfort, the following are advised:
◆ close-fitting sleeves and cuffs to avoid catching fabric in the wheels;
◆ longer-length skirts for a woman so that they fall easily over her knees when she is seated;
◆ short coats or jackets so that the person is not sitting on them; long coats can also get caught in the wheels;
◆ low-heeled, well-fitting shoes with nonslip soles, because these are less likely to slip off the footrests;
◆ short scarves that can be tied easily so that they don't get caught in the wheels.

SIMPLE FASTENINGS

Snaps These are fastened by simply pressing together both halves. Use instead of buttons.

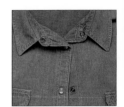

Large buttons Small buttons can be difficult to grip. Choose garments with large buttons or replace small ones and widen the buttonholes.

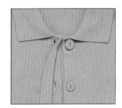

Drawstring waist Choose garments that have an elasticized waist. A drawstring is easy to tie and untie and an elasticated waist is more comfortable.

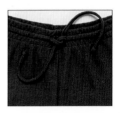

Velcro This consists of two nylon surfaces that stick to each other when pressed together. Replace buttons with velcro and resew them over the buttonholes.

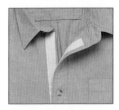

Invisible zipper pull The catch is attached through the hole in the zipper tag. The zipper is pulled by the loop, which can then be tucked away.

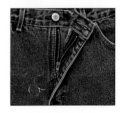

CHAPTER 10

BLADDER &
BOWEL CONTROL

Problems that affect the bladder and bowel range from
incontinence, constipation, and diarrhea, to abnormalities of
the urinary and lower digestive tracts.

INCONTINENCE

Looking after a person who has lost control of the
bladder or bowel – a condition known as incontinence – is
possibly one of the most difficult tasks for any caregiver.
Incontinence occurs when illness, injury, or degeneration disturbs
normal bladder or bowel function, leading to the involuntary
discharge of urine or feces. It is a distressing and embarrassing
condition that may lead to the incontinent person isolating
himself and trying to cope alone. The problem must be addressed
to find ways to allow the person independence and privacy. In
many cases, it is possible to discover a medical solution.

MEDICAL TREATMENTS

Medical advice should always be sought for bladder
and bowel problems. Solutions range from prescribed drugs to
treatment that diverts the passage of urine or feces. These
treatments are now very refined and, with the proper care, can
significantly enhance the person's quality of life.

MINOR CONDITIONS

Bladder and bowel conditions, which include urinary problems, constipation, and diarrhea, may be symptoms of an underlying illness, an infection, or a treatment. If your relative complains of any change in his bladder or bowel movements, such as discomfort or discoloration, or he has any difficulty in going to the toilet, you should always seek medical advice.

URINATION AND DEFECATION

Someone who is healthy will pass urine and feces naturally.

How urine is passed:
◆ The bladder stores urine produced in the kidneys.

◆ As the bladder fills, nerve impulses signal to the brain that the bladder is full and must be emptied.

◆ The urine is passed – and discharged – through a tube (the *urethra*) connected to the bladder.

How feces are passed:
◆ Digestion takes place as food passes from the stomach to the small intestine.

◆ Any nutrients are absorbed into the bloodstream; what remains passes into the large intestine.

◆ This waste matter (*feces*), which is no longer required by the body, is stored in the large intestine before being expelled via the rectum.

RECOGNITION AND TREATMENTS

Once you recognize that there is a problem, you can identify possible causes and explore treatments.

WHAT TO DO FOR URINARY PROBLEMS
Your relative may have an infection if passing urine causes stinging and discomfort, or if the urine:
◆ is dark or cloudy in color, or contains blood;
◆ has a particularly pungent smell;
◆ is being passed in small quantities frequently.
Seek medical help Your relative's physician may need to prescribe medication to treat the infection if it is the cause of the urinary problem.

WHAT TO DO FOR CONSTIPATION
This condition occurs when the person has failed to open his bowels as normal. There may be an obstruction, or the waste matter (*feces*) may have become dry, making it difficult to pass.
Seek medical help A doctor may prescribe laxatives, suppositories, or, in severe cases, an enema.
Encourage toilet use Encourage your relative to use the toilet regularly, even though he may be reluctant to do so because his bowel movements are painful.
Adapt the diet Make sure he eats a balanced diet (*see pages 61–63*) and drinks plenty of fluids.

WHAT TO DO FOR DIARRHEA
When a person passes liquid feces at frequent intervals, the condition is known as diarrhea.
Seek medical help Consult a physician, especially if the person is elderly or sick.
Adapt the diet Give your relative plenty of fluids, including water. Abstaining from solid food for 24 hours may also help relieve diarrhea.

INCONTINENCE

THIS CAN BE URINARY OR FECAL, although the latter is rare. Incontinence is a medical condition, but a person who has toilet "accidents" may be diagnosed as incontinent because he cannot cope with the normal sequence of events involved in going to the toilet. If your relative is incontinent, consult a healthcare professional to find an effective way to manage and treat the problem.

CAUSES AND TREATMENTS

CAUSE	WHAT HAPPENS	TREATMENT
Enlarged prostate gland	◆ The enlarged prostate gland blocks the passage of urine. The bladder fills up and then involuntarily releases an overflow of urine.	◆ Insertion of a catheter. ◆ Surgery or other treatment to remove the prostate gland.
Weak muscle tone	◆ The muscles that control the passing of urine or feces become weak so that urine (and, rarely, feces) are passed involuntarily after coughing or mild exercise. This is stress incontinence.	◆ Kegel exercises. ◆ Toilet routine. ◆ Surgery.
Infection	◆ Someone who has an infection may have a strong urge to urinate followed by an involuntary emptying of the bladder. Passing urine may be painful, causing a burning sensation.	◆ Medication to treat the cause of infection. ◆ Sufficient fluid intake.
Damage to the nervous system	◆ If the nervous system is damaged, the person may be unable to recognize his need to use the toilet.	◆ Relearning control. ◆ Use of toilet aids. ◆ Insertion of a catheter.
Constipation	◆ Feces become impacted in the rectum (see opposite); liquid feces may seep out. In some cases, the resulting pressure on the bladder may lead to urinary incontinence.	◆ A high-fiber diet and sufficient fluids. ◆ Drugs, such as laxatives. ◆ Regular enemas, if condition persists.
Immobility and dementia	◆ For both conditions, a person may have normal bladder and bowel function but be unable to get to the toilet in time, or need help once there. With dementia, he may also be unable to express his need to go to the toilet.	◆ Toilet routine. ◆ Use of toilet aids (with supervision for someone who has dementia).

PROMOTING CONTINENCE

IF YOUR RELATIVE cannot be treated medically (*see page 115*), he may have to rely on the use of aids (*see pages 112–14*). However, by pinpointing why the incontinence occurs, you may be able to establish a toilet routine and address any mental or physical problems that are causing the difficulties. This may help your relative regain continence, or, at least alleviate the problem.

PINPOINTING AND SOLVING THE PROBLEM

The chart below is designed to help you identify the cause of the problem and give you guidance on how to help your relative to be continent. However, always seek the advice of a healthcare professional, such as a physician, nurse practioner, or continence adviser, as soon as the problem begins.

HOW TO HELP AN INCONTINENT PERSON		
PROBLEM	AIM	WHAT YOU CAN DO
A paralyzed person He may be physically unable to recognize that he needs to use the toilet.	To recognize that urine or feces need to be passed.	**Encourage toilet use** To establish a toilet routine, make sure that your relative goes to the toilet, or is taken there, every 2–3 hours. **Establish a pattern** Note times that the incontinence occurs and, if a pattern emerges, prompt him about half an hour before these times. **Use reminders** Set an alarm clock or kitchen timer to ring when he usually needs the toilet.
A person with dementia He may know when he needs the toilet, but be unable to express this need. **An immobile person** He may be unable to get to the toilet.	To know where the toilet is and be able to get there.	**Deal with confusion** Redecorating or moving to a new house may disorientate a confused person. Tell the person where the toilet is or put up signs until he is more confident of his whereabouts. **Think about location** Ensure that an immobile person's living and sleeping quarters are near the toilet. If necessary, put up handrails to help him get there, and make sure the route is free of obstacles. If he is unable to go to the toilet by himself, take him every 2–3 hours or obtain an aid for occasional use (*see page 114*).
A physically impaired person He may have difficulty undoing his clothes.	To undo or remove necessary clothing easily.	**Provide practical clothes** Make sure that your relative wears clothes that are easy to remove; avoid small buttons or difficult fastenings (*see page 106*). Don't leave him in pajamas all day; if he feels he is not trusted, the incontinence may get worse .

GETTING HELP

Only one out of every ten caregivers looking after an incontinent person asks for help. Do not be afraid to use the resources available to you, and do not hesitate to find out if you qualify for financial help.

SPECIALIST ADVICE

Ask the physician or nurse practitioner to refer your relative to a continence adviser, who will be able to assess his needs and advise you both accordingly. Seek advice from specialist organizations, such as National Association for Continence (*see page 175*).

INCONTINENCE AIDS

There is a wide variety of incontinence aids (*see pages 112–15*) available that will make it easier for you and your relative to deal with the problem. For example, specialized bedding will reduce the amount of washing you have to do and add to your relative's comfort. Some aids, such as incontinence pads, may be provided free of charge; find out what is available and suitable from a continence adviser.

LAUNDRY

Continual washing can add to the burden of caring for an incontinent person. Find out if your local authority offers a laundry service.

FINANCIAL

Find out if you are eligible for benefits to cover the expense associated with incontinence (*see pages 164–68*).

ADAPTING AN INCONTINENT PERSON'S DIET

In some cases, adapting your relative's diet and fluid intake can help control incontinence.

Food A high-fiber diet can help to prevent constipation, which may be the cause of fecal incontinence.

Fluid Limiting drinks in the evening may help if the urinary incontinence tends to occur at night. Do not, however, try to deal with urinary incontinence by limiting fluid intake during the day. It is essential to your relative's health that he drinks sufficient fluids.

COPING EMOTIONALLY

Incontinence can be a very difficult problem to cope with and, sadly, it is one of the main reasons why people give up their caregiving role. The problem is aggravated when the person does not admit to the problem and tries to cover up accidents by hiding dirty clothes, or when he appears to be incontinent on purpose. Before you can begin to deal with the problem, whatever its cause, it is important for both of you to be honest about how you feel.

Your feelings It is very normal to feel angry and disgusted by having to deal with incontinence. If you are finding it difficult to cope, seek help (*see left*). Trying to cope alone will not be beneficial for either you or your relative.

Your relative's feelings It is very likely to be embarrassing and frustrating for your relative if he has to rely on you because he is unable to carry out these most basic functions. Allow him as much privacy and independence as possible. Encourage him to talk about it and try to be understanding.

INCONTINENCE AIDS

THERE IS A RANGE OF AIDS to help with incontinence. Ask to see a continence adviser, who will be able to assess the extent of your relative's problem, taking his age and mental and physical condition into account. This specialist will also be able to give you advice on the devices most likely to help your relative, and will provide information on available medical benefits.

ALARM CLOCK

An alarm clock is useful if your relative does not recognize his need to go to the toilet. To establish a routine, set the alarm to go off every 2–3 hours as a reminder that it is time to use the toilet.

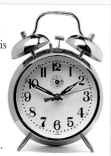

COMFORT AID

Commode ring This circular, air-filled ring can be used on most commodes (*see page 114*). It is an aid to comfort and is especially useful if your relative is suffering from pressure sores (*see page 96*).

Commode

Commode ring

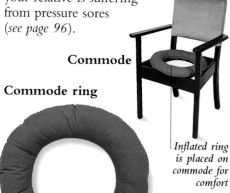

Inflated ring is placed on commode for comfort

— *Be careful not to overinflate*

PADS AND PANTS

Incontinence pads There are designs for men and women, and a variety of sizes and absorbency levels (double for maximum absorbency). They can be used with or without special briefs. The pad, which works on the same principle as a diaper, will absorb moisture and keep the wearer's skin dry.

Male pad

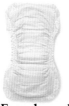

Female pad

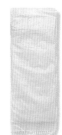

Double pad

Incontinence pants Special briefs are available that have a pouch for an incontinence pad. The pad should be positioned well to the front for a man and farther back for a woman. Encourage your relative to insert the pad himself, if he is capable. There are also washable, reusable briefs that have a built-in pad.

Waterproof pouch for pad

BEDDING FOR AN INCONTINENT PERSON

There is a wide variety of incontinence products available, from mattress and pillow protectors to incontinence sheets. There are different degrees of absorbency to suit the level of incontinence. You may not need all the items shown below; a continence adviser will recommend those most suitable for your relative. Whenever possible, choose bedding that is easy to wash and dry. A mattress protector may make some people sweat excessively; discontinue use if this happens. For your relative's comfort, and to prevent sores developing, always change wet bedding as quickly as possible.

PROTECTING BEDDING

1 Place a fitted water-proof protector over the mattress.

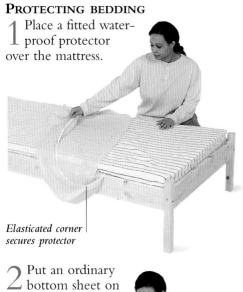

Elasticated corner secures protector

2 Put an ordinary bottom sheet on top of the protector and tuck it in securely.

Place bottom sheet over mattress protector

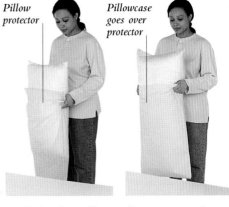

Pillow protector   *Pillowcase goes over protector*

3 Strip the pillow of its cover and replace it with a waterproof protector. Put an ordinary pillowcase over the protector.

4 Place an absorbent bed protector over the bottom sheet.

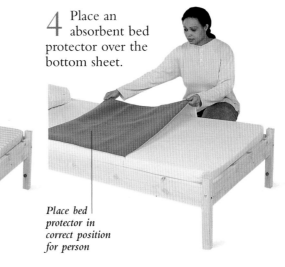

Place bed protector in correct position for person

TOILET AIDS

IF YOUR RELATIVE IS IMMOBILE OR BEDRIDDEN, he may benefit from the use of a toilet aid, such as a urinal, commode, or bedpan. These aids will help reduce the risk of him having an "accident," and give him a degree of independence when he is using the toilet.

USING SPECIAL TOILETS

When your relative wants to use a urinal, commode, or bedpan, make sure:
◆ he is able to unbutton or remove the necessary clothing easily;
◆ there is toilet paper within reach;
◆ he can be left in private, if possible.

After using the toilet, establish a way for your relative to communicate to you that he has finished, then:
◆ help him clean himself, if he is unable to do this on his own;
◆ make sure he washes his hands;
◆ wash the equipment (*see page 57*);
◆ wash your hands (*see page 56*).

Urinals These are mainly used by men, but the pan type can be used by women, and is good for wheelchair use.
How to help Encourage your relative to use it alone, but if he is unable to do so, help him. It is difficult for a man to use a urinal lying down, so he may need to sit, supported on the edge of the bed.

Commode

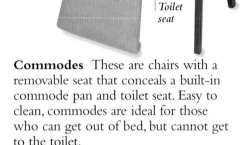

Removable padded seat cover

Toilet seat

Commodes These are chairs with a removable seat that conceals a built-in commode pan and toilet seat. Easy to clean, commodes are ideal for those who can get out of bed, but cannot get to the toilet.
How to help Help the person onto the commode, and give him as much privacy as his condition allows.

Bedpans These are used for a person who cannot get out of bed. The wedge-shaped fracture type is particularly easy to use, allowing the person to slide backward and lift himself onto it.
How to help If it is a steel pan, make sure it is warm and dry. Ask him to raise himself, or help him to do this, then slide the bedpan underneath him. Provide a man with a urinal as well (*see left*).

Fracture bedpan

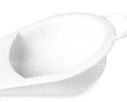

Wedge-shaped for easier positioning

Female urinal

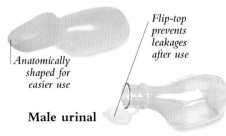

Anatomically shaped for easier use

Flip-top prevents leakages after use

Male urinal

MEDICAL TREATMENTS

IT MAY BE NECESSARY for a person with bladder and bowel problems to be fitted with a device that allows urine or feces to be passed and collected through a different channel: a catheter for someone with urinary incontinence, or a stoma with a bag for someone who has a disease of the digestive tract (*see page 116*). If properly maintained, these can enhance the person's quality of life.

CATHETER CARE

As part of the medical treatment for a bladder problem or as a last resort for untreatable incontinence, a tube (*catheter*) may be inserted into the bladder to drain urine. The tube is then attached to a collecting bag strapped to the person's leg or waist.

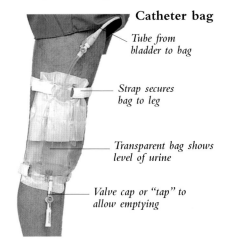

Catheter bag

Tube from bladder to bag

Strap secures bag to leg

Transparent bag shows level of urine

Valve cap or "tap" to allow emptying

LOOKING AFTER THE CATHETER

Most catheters are inserted into the bladder and left in place. The person will be shown when and how to empty the bag. The tube is replaced periodically by a physician or nurse practitioner. People with intermittent incontinence, such as those with multiple sclerosis, may be taught to insert a catheter. To prevent infection, the person should wash the area around the catheter every day with

soap and water, and drink plenty of fluids. You should know the washing and emptying procedures because you may have to help your relative.

EMPTYING A CATHETER BAG

The bag should be emptied about every four hours or when it is more than two-thirds full.

Draining the bag The cap at the bottom of the bag is opened and the urine is drained into a container kept for this purpose. The urine is flushed down the toilet. If the bag is supplied separately, it may have to be changed. Follow instructions carefully and wear gloves to minimize the risk of infection.

Checking the tube After emptying, the tube that leads from the catheter to the bag should be checked to make sure it is not kinked or blocked.

DEALING WITH COMPLICATIONS

A catheter may cause a urinary infection. If your relative complains of a burning sensation when urinating or has cloudy urine, it may indicate an infection. Always seek medical help. If the catheter actually comes out, no attempt should be made to reinsert it because this may seriously damage the bladder or urethra. If any complications arise, consult a continence adviser or the physician.

STOMA CARE

When the digestive tract is diseased or damaged in some way, or it is not possible for the person to pass feces normally, surgery may be necessary.
The stoma Part of the large intestine (a *colostomy*) or small intestine (an *ileostomy*) can be brought out onto the abdomen to form an opening (*stoma*). The size of the stoma may vary in size and color. It will be quite red and swollen at first, but may become smaller and turn pink. A specialized bag is fitted over the stoma to collect feces. A person who has a temporary stoma may still be able to pass feces normally.

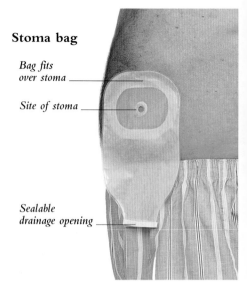

Stoma bag

Bag fits over stoma

Site of stoma

Sealable drainage opening

SPECIALIST ADVICE

Before and after surgery, the person will be cared for by a enterostomal therapist. The best position for the stoma will be discussed, although it may not always be possible to decide on the site before surgery. The therapist will also provide information about the operation and advice on aftercare. For additional information, contact the United Ostomy Association (*see page 176*).

AFTERCARE

A stoma should not prevent a person from leading a normal life. Stoma bags are very well designed and are not noticeable even under shorts or a swimsuit. If the correct aftercare is given, normal bowel movement should return, enabling the person to resume a full and active life. The person will need to follow specialist advice on changing the bag, skin care, and diet. As the caregiver, you can help by making sure that there is an adequate supply of bags, which are usually prescribed.

Stoma bag The enterostomal therapist will show your relative how to change the bag (*see below*). There are different designs available.
Skin care Your relative will be shown how to wash and dry around the stoma and how to identify an infection.
Diet Advice will be provided on identifying and cutting out foods that cause problems.

CHANGING A STOMA BAG

The bag is usually changed twice a day. Allow your relative privacy, and make sure that he has everything he requires. For the procedure he will need a bowl of warm water, soap, a towel, a replacement bag, and a disposal bag, which should be provided.
The normal procedure is as follows:
♦ the stoma bag is removed and placed in the disposal bag;
♦ the stoma and surrounding area is cleaned with warm water and soap, and dried thoroughly;
♦ the new bag is attached.

CHAPTER 11

HOME FROM THE HOSPITAL

Your role as a caregiver may begin when your relative is discharged from the hospital. Before this happens, the hospital should ensure that you have all the resources you need to provide adequate aftercare.

AFTERCARE

Planning aftercare will be easier if you find out as much as possible about your relative's condition and the type of hospital treatment she has undergone. If you are caring for your relative full-time, you may need professional assistance or part-time help from a volunteer caregiver. In some situations, the special facilities and services of a day center may provide the psychological and physical care your relative needs, and can also offer you advice, support, and some relief from your role.

REHABILITATION AND CONVALESCENCE

A major operation or illness may have a profound emotional effect on your relative, especially if she has restricted mobility and is dependent on others for the first time in her adult life. She may also take time to adjust to being back at home, particularly if she has been in the hospital for a long period of time.

LEAVING THE HOSPITAL

YOU AND YOUR RELATIVE should be consulted from the outset by the hospital about arrangements for discharge; these details may even begin before your relative goes into the hospital or when she is admitted. As the main caregiver, you will be told when to pick her up from the hospital, how to care for her at home, how to administer medicines, and what follow-up visits are required.

YOUR RELATIVE'S RIGHTS

The welfare of both your relative and yourself is paramount in the discharge procedure. Your relative has certain rights according to the Patient's Bill of Rights (*see pages 172–73*). Each of you has the right to complain if you are dissatisfied.

Hospital staff First, speak to the nurse in charge or, if you do not find that effective, to the hospital manager.

Complaints procedure If you are still not satisfied, make a formal complaint, following the hospital's procedures.

Specialist help Seek help from the ward staff, your physician, or your area agency on aging (*see pages 176–77*) on how to make a complaint. The Patient's Association and your state long-term care ombudsman will also be able to advise you on the proper procedure for filing a complaint.

BEFORE YOUR RELATIVE IS DISCHARGED

Hospital staff should discharge a patient only when they are satisfied that there is someone to care for her at home. They should always consult the patient about this, and you, as the main caregiver. You will need to liaise with various members of staff, such as the nurse in charge, the social worker, and the physician, in planning your relative's discharge and aftercare. You should agree to allow her to come home only when you are totally satisfied with the arrangements.

QUESTIONS YOU SHOULD ASK THE HOSPITAL STAFF

Do not be afraid to ask questions about your relative's condition and the type of care she needs. Find out:
♦ what medicines she needs, how frequently they are required, and how they should be administered;
♦ whether the medicines or treatments have any side effects; if so, how these should be managed;
♦ how to carry out specific moving and handling maneuvers, on your own or with help;
♦ how to cope if anything goes wrong.

PREPARATIONS THE HOSPITAL STAFF SHOULD MAKE

Before your relative leaves the hospital, a member of the staff will consult you, the main caregiver, and tell you when to collect her. They will also:
♦ inform the physician and nurse practitioner of the discharge, and explain her condition and likely needs;
♦ order the medicines for her immediate aftercare;
♦ arrange any specialized aftercare services, such as physical therapy or occupational therapy;
♦ if necessary, arrange transportation home;
♦ give you instructions regarding the aftercare and follow-up visits to the hospital;
♦ tell your relative when she can return to work.

PREPARING THE HOME

BEFORE YOUR RELATIVE LEAVES THE HOSPITAL, you need to ensure that you have the necessary resources and skills to provide adequate care. Find out from the nurse practitioner or the physician exactly what is required of you. Once you are sure that you can undertake the caregiving role, you can make preparations for your relative's return home. (*See also* Being a Caregiver, *pages 13–28*).

PREPARING YOURSELF FOR CAREGIVING

Before you decide that you can provide adequate care, ask yourself the following questions:
◆ Do I fully understand why my relative was admitted to the hospital and what treatments she received?
◆ Am I physically and mentally capable of caring for my relative day and night?
◆ Who do I turn to in an emergency? Do I have the telephone numbers of the physician (or on-call hospital doctor) and Eldercare Locator (*see page 174*)?
◆ Do I have enough support from other people, such as a friend, relative, or volunteer caregiver, where necessary, to help look after my relative?
◆ What effect will the caregiving role have on other members of my household?
◆ Is the home sufficiently equipped? For example, are special toilet facilities, or any special aids, such as a wheelchair, needed?
If you are unsure about any of the above, you should speak to the nursing staff or your relative's physician before agreeing to take on the caregiving role.

PRACTICAL ARRANGEMENTS AT HOME

Before your relative leaves the hospital, you should make thorough preparations at home.
Preparing her room Make sure that your relative's bedroom is clean and comfortable and that it is not too hot or too cold. The layout of the room should be practical, with bedside items at hand (*see page 52*).
Preparing a meal Have a light meal ready since she may be hungry, but bear in mind dietary restrictions.
Organizing visitors Stagger visits from family and friends. Talk to your relative to see if she feels up to seeing people, bearing in mind that she may feel tired.

PROLONGED ILLNESSES

Caring for someone with a prolonged illness, such as cancer or kidney disease, can be particularly difficult. Your relative will require a lot of emotional support, particularly if she is undergoing intensive treatment, such as chemotherapy or dialysis. The closer you are to someone, the more difficult it can be, so it is advisable to seek outside support.

Support groups
Various organizations such as Alzheimer's Association or the American Parkinson's Disease Association (*see pages 175–76*), offer advice and support to the affected person, family, and friends. A support group for caregivers, such as National Caregiving Association (*see page 174*), may be able to put you and your relative in contact with others in a similar situation.

REHABILITATION

AFTER YOUR RELATIVE COMES OUT OF THE HOSPITAL, she may not be able to carry out some day-to-day tasks, such as having a bath or cooking for herself. You will need to assess the level of help she requires but allow her to be as independent as possible. She may also have been prescribed treatment, such as physical therapy, to take place at home, a day center, or the hospital.

EMOTIONAL SUPPORT

Try to be sensitive to how your relative is feeling, particularly if she has experienced a major operation or an illness that required lengthy treatment. If she has had a life-changing operation or illness, she may benefit from outside support, such as counseling, to overcome any anxiety.

Gathering information
Find out as much as you can from the hospital staff about your relative's illness and the likely effects of the treatment she has undergone.

Seeking support
Various support groups have been established to help people care for specific conditions. Ask your physician or nurse practitioner to put you in touch with one for help and advice, or telephone the relevant organization directly for information (see pages 174–76).

REESTABLISHING A DAILY ROUTINE

You will need to establish a routine that will ease your relative back into home life and help her regain her health. Her daily timetable should be based on the information supplied by the hospital staff and on her individual needs. Bear in mind the following points, when working out a routine:
- how much rest she needs;
- what type of diet she requires;
- what she is physically capable of doing;
- what medication she takes;
- any specially devised aftercare program, such as physical therapy exercises (see opposite);
- follow-up treatments at the hospital and check-up visits from her physician and nurse practitioner.

HELPING YOUR RELATIVE TO ADJUST

Once your relative is home, bear in mind her physical and emotional needs. She is likely to be too weak to carry out all the daily activities she undertook before going into the hospital. She may feel insecure or even confused about being out of the routine of the hospital ward. Patience is required while she adjusts to the new location and a different way of doing things.
Rest Encourage her to take things slowly. She should rest for at least an hour in the afternoon, and catnap whenever she is tired.
Exercise If she is mobile, encourage her to take gentle exercise, even if it is only walking around indoors.
Companionship Try not to leave her alone for long periods, because she may feel isolated after being in a busy hospital ward. Although it is good for her to receive visitors, make sure she is ready for this. If possible, find time to talk to her about how she feels, and be encouraging and reassuring.

TREATMENTS AND THERAPIES

Rehabilitation means restoring an individual to normal function after a disease or injury. This process can take a long time and may require your relative to undergo regular treatments and therapies.
◆ As part of her treatment, your relative may be shown exercises that she can carry out herself.
◆ As the main caregiver, you may be taught simple techniques that you can regularly use at home.
◆ A qualified therapist might visit your home to treat your relative.
◆ Your relative may go for treatment at a day center, which might also be linked to a hospital.

DAY CENTERS

Many day centers are specially equipped for elderly and disabled people and those recovering from an accident or operation. Treatment may be carried out at one of these centers if, for example, the use of specialized equipment or the skills of trained staff are required. Day centers also allow your relative to meet people who have similar needs, and give you, the caregiver, the chance to have a break.

THE RANGE OF THERAPIES

Following a thorough assessment of your relative's condition, the most effective treatment is prescribed.
Physical therapy This is a combination of exercises prescribed by a physical therapist for the patient's individual needs. The exercises are used to strengthen and heal parts of the body in conjunction with heat treatments or ultrasound, for example.
Hydrotherapy These are exercise sessions that take place in a swimming pool. Water reduces the pull of gravity on the injured part of the body, making movement easier and thereby reducing pain.
Occupational therapy This form of therapy helps a person to relearn everyday skills that have been lost as a result of illness or injury, such as dressing, bathing, and preparing meals. It is particularly useful for stroke patients or for those who are otherwise disabled.
Speech–language therapy This range of exercises is designed to help someone overcome a language or speech difficulty (*see page 39*).

PHYSICAL THERAPY AT HOME

A physical therapist will demonstrate techniques to help your relative strengthen her limbs and improve dexterity.

Hand therapy
Special items, such as putty balls, can be manipulated by hand to improve dexterity and strengthen wrist and hand movement.

Limb therapy This is effective for someone who has restricted movement. A common exercise may require you, the caregiver, to hold the limb (at the wrist and elbow, or ankle and knee) and move it upward, exercising all the joints without pushing beyond the natural movement of the limb.

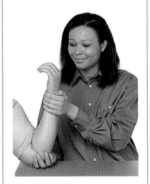

Physical therapy exercises You can help your relative by carrying out gentle limb therapy.

HOSPITAL DAY TREATMENTS

ADVANCES IN MEDICAL TECHNOLOGY have helped to speed up treatments, allowing a patient to be admitted to the hospital as an outpatient. In some situations a general anesthetic may be given, while other procedures may be carried out under local anesthetic or sedation. You and your relative will be told what the treatment involves and what aftercare is required.

WHY DAY TREATMENTS ARE CARRIED OUT

Many disorders can be treated in a hospital's outpatient department. Some day procedures are also required to investigate a condition to see whether an operation is needed or to give treatment following an operation. Understanding the treatment will help you to provide the best aftercare.

A GUIDE TO THE TESTS, TREATMENTS, AND AFTEREFFECTS

TREATMENT	WHAT HAPPENS	AFTEREFFECTS
Barium X ray	Barium is a substance that shows up on an X ray. The patient swallows a barium "meal," which is then x-rayed (as it progresses through the intestinal tract) to investigate the bowel and rectum. Barium may also be given as an enema.	White feces may be passed. The patient may become constipated.
MRI scan	Magnetic Resonance Imaging (MRI) uses magnetic fields and radiowaves to make detailed cross-sectional pictures of the head and body, which are translated by a computer into high-quality images. The patient will be asked to remove any metal objects, and to lie very still on a bed that moves through the tunnel-shaped scanner. She will hear instructions from the nurse through headphones.	The scan is painless and there are no aftereffects.
Keyhole surgery (for example, laparascopy)	For some conditions, this is an alternative to major surgery. Tiny viewing instruments (*scopes*) are passed through small incisions in the body, then manipulated to examine and remove tissue and tumors. Typical procedures are treatment of some hernias, and removing cartilage from a knee joint.	There will be some pain and discomfort, but recuperation is swift because the surgery is relatively minimal.

A Guide to the Treatments and Aftereffects

Treatment	What Happens	Aftereffects
Chemotherapy	This treatment of cancer or infection may involve the injection of drugs through a vein in order to destroy abnormal cells. The first sessions usually take place in a cancer (*oncology*) unit; thereafter, they may be continued in an outpatient department and sometimes at home. In other instances, the treatment may only involve taking medication in tablet form.	Vomiting (*see page 70*) and diarrhea (*see page 108*) can leave the patient feeling weak and tired. Hair loss may occur.
Radiation therapy	This treats cancer through special X rays directed at the affected part of the body to destroy the diseased or unwanted tissue. Radiation therapy may be used together with chemotherapy to treat some cancers.	Vomiting (*see page 70*) and diarrhea (*see page 108*) can leave the patient feeling weak and tired.
Kidney dialysis	A procedure designed to remove harmful toxic elements from the blood and excess fluid from the body as treatment for kidney failure. Nurses or technicians operate a dialysis machine and can train the caregiver and relative to do the procedure at home.	Hunger, thirst, and occasional confusion.
Gastroscopy	Long, flexible viewing instruments (*gastroscopes*) are passed through the mouth and used to investigate conditions of the stomach. A doctor views the stomach lining and makes a diagnosis.	Patients often complain of a sore throat and/or gas for a day or two after this procedure.
Cystoscopy	A method of examining the bladder: a viewing instrument (*cystoscope*) is inserted into the urethra to investigate blood in the urine and other related conditions.	Discomfort may last for 24 hours and some blood may be passed. Drinking plenty of fluids helps prevent infection and makes it easier to pass urine.
Casts	Someone with a dislocation or broken bone may need day treatment to change a cast. Plaster of paris or acrylic is molded and shaped while wet; once dry and rigid, it supports the injured part while it heals.	Check circulation in the fingers or toes. If they are cold, blue, or tingle ("pins and needles"), seek medical advice.

CONVALESCENCE

RECOVERY FROM AN ILLNESS OR OPERATION may leave your relative immobile and restricted in what she is able to do. This often leads to boredom, frustration, and depression. You may be able to help by encouraging pastimes that will keep her busy, and her mind active. These activities can help her focus on regaining good health and maximum independence.

ITEMS THAT AID RECOVERY

There are many aids on the market that can help your relative to overcome physical difficulties.

Book stand A light, folding book stand can be used by a weak person to hold a book.

Magnifier This is a visual aid that helps someone with impaired vision to read and carry out detailed work.

Knitting machine This is designed to enable a disabled person to knit with one hand.

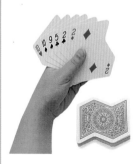

Crooked cards Useful for someone who cannot grip.

RECREATIONAL ACTIVITIES

As soon as your relative is well enough, try to introduce activities that encourage a more positive state of mind. Hobbies, games, and gentle exercise will greatly improve the later stages of recovery by providing mental and physical stimulation, offering a welcome diversion from immobility, and helping to boost confidence.

HOBBIES AND INTERESTS

As your relative begins to make progress, incorporate a hobby or interest into her daily routine. If she is an elderly or disabled person, she may be able to resume a hobby with the use of appropriate aids. Equipment such as a kneeling frame, for example, allows a gardener to lower and raise herself with ease.

PLAYING GAMES

Playing cards or board games, and doing crossword and jigsaw puzzles, are pastimes that you can enjoy together. These activities can help keep your relative's mind alert, lift her spirits, and encourage gentle motion of the upper body.

GENTLE EXERCISE

Encourage your relative to walk very short distances, then build on this according to her progress. If she is not able to walk, a short car ride will at least give her an opportunity to leave the house.

HANDICRAFTS

Crafts, such as knitting, painting, and model-making, are absorbing for those who like working with their hands. These activities can be very therapeutic and are ideal for those whose mobility is restricted.

CHAPTER 12

CAREGIVING SKILLS

Part of your role may involve caring for your
relative while he has a long- or short-term illness.
As with all aspects of caring, looking after a sick person at
home requires common sense. Your primary aims are to make
sure that your relative is comfortable and, where possible, to
help alleviate any painful or distressing symptoms.
For example, if he can't get out of bed, something as simple as
keeping the room clean and well ventilated may help make him
feel better, or if he has a condition that causes breathing
difficulties, you may be able to help by making
sure that he is in a comfortable position.

PRACTICAL SKILLS

The pages that follow give you a basic
understanding of the practical skills you need to look after
someone who is sick: how to take someone's temperature and
measure his pulse rate, how to relieve uncomfortable symptoms,
and what information to record and pass on to the doctor.
There is also a guide to the type
of medication that is likely to be prescribed and how it
should be administered. If you are unable to deal with any aspect
of this type of caregiving, are concerned about your relative's
symptoms, or are unclear on any aspects of his medication, always
seek the advice of a healthcare professional, such as
a physician or registered nurse.

Temperature Changes

A HEALTHY BODY MAINTAINS a constant temperature of between 96.8 and 98.6°F (36–37°C) by achieving a balance between the heat it produces and the heat it loses. If this balance is disturbed, a body temperature outside the normal range will result. This is often a sign of illness, so you will need to seek medical help and, in the meantime, try to alleviate any symptoms.

Recognizing an Abnormal Body Temperature

A body temperature below 96.8°F (36°C) or above 98.6°F (37°C) may have clear signs (*see below*). Fast or slow pulse and breathing rates may also indicate an abnormal temperature (*see page 128*).

Signs of a very low temperature
The person will feel cold and may be:
◆ shivering
◆ pale
◆ confused

Signs of a high temperature
The person will feel hot and may:
◆ have flushed cheeks
◆ be sweating
◆ be shivering

Why changes occur
An extreme rise or fall in temperature can occur if the body's heat regulating mechanism fails.

Low temperature A drop in temperature below 95°F (35°C) (*hypothermia*) occurs when the body loses more heat than it can produce. This can occur outdoors in very cold weather conditions, and indoors if preventive measures are not taken (*see page 129*).

High temperature This is part of the body's natural defense mechanism (*see page 56*) for fighting infection. The increase in temperature above 98.6°F (37°C) (*pyrexia*) helps destroy many bacteria and viruses.

Thermometers

Mercury and digital thermometers are the most commonly used. The former indicates temperature by means of a mercury level, the latter by a digital reading.

Temperature
◆ 96.8–98.6°F (36–37°C) = normal
◆ above 98.6°F (37°C) = fever
◆ below 95°F (35°C) = hypothermia

Mercury thermometer

Mercury level

Normal temperature range

A reading outside the 96.8–98.6°F (36–37°C) range can be a danger sign

Digital reading

Digital thermometer

TAKING A TEMPERATURE

Taking the temperature orally is the most common and effective method. If, for any reason, this is not possible (*see right*), the reading should be taken under the armpit (*see page 128*). You should, however, let the physician know that you used this method because it is less accurate. You should never take the temperature via the rectum; this method should only be carried out by a doctor or nurse and is rarely necessary.

WHEN NOT TO USE THE MOUTH

Taking the temperature by mouth is not safe or effective if someone:
◆ is unconscious;
◆ is confused or mentally impaired;
◆ is a baby, or a child under age six;
◆ is suffering from a jaw injury;
◆ is susceptible to convulsions;
◆ has a cough or blocked nose;
◆ has recently had a hot or cold drink.

TAKING A TEMPERATURE BY MOUTH

1 Clean the thermometer by rinsing it in cold water and drying it with a clean cloth. If you are using a mercury thermometer, shake it until the mercury level is at the bottom of the scale. If you are using a digital thermometer, clean it, switch it on, then wait for the screen to go blank.

Place thermometer under her tongue

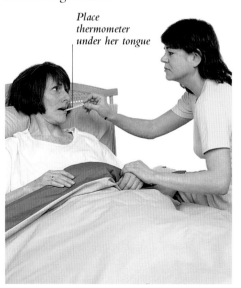

2 Place the thermometer under the person's tongue and ask her to close her lips securely to hold it in place.

3 Leave a mercury thermometer in the person's mouth for three to five minutes. Leave a digital thermometer until it beeps.

Hold thermometer steady and in a good light

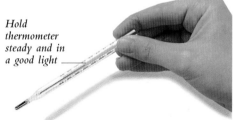

4 Remove the thermometer and record the temperature by noting the mercury level or digital reading.

5 Shake the mercury back down or turn the digital thermometer off.

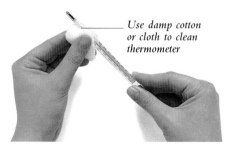

Use damp cotton or cloth to clean thermometer

6 Wipe the thermometer clean and return it to its case.

TAKING A TEMPERATURE UNDER THE ARMPIT

1 Rinse the thermometer in cold water and dry it with a clean cloth. Shake the mercury down to the bottom of the scale or, if you are using a digital thermometer, switch it on.

2 Make sure the thermometer and the skin under the armpit are dry. Ask the person to keep still.

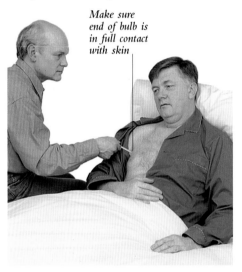

Make sure end of bulb is in full contact with skin

3 Place the thermometer in the person's armpit and ask him to fold his forearm across his chest.

4 Leave a mercury thermometer in place for three to five minutes. Leave a digital thermometer until it beeps.

5 Record the temperature by noting the mercury level or digital reading.

6 Shake the mercury back down or turn the digital thermometer off. Wipe the thermometer clean and return it to its case.

BREATHING AND PULSE RATES

While taking a temperature, you should check your relative's breathing and pulse rates because an increase or decrease in these can also indicate a temperature change. The information can then be recorded and given to the physician, along with the temperature reading.

Monitor breathing At rest, a person breathes in and out (one respiration) about 16 times per minute. Anything above or below this may accompany a high or low temperature. Count your relative's breaths per minute and note your findings for the physician. To get a more accurate measure, do not tell him that you are monitoring his breathing.

Check the pulse The pulse is the "wave" that courses through the body each time the heart pumps blood into the circulatory system. The normal pulse rate for a person at rest is between 60–80 beats per minute; anything above or below this level, and any change in the strength of the pulse, may accompany a high or low temperature.

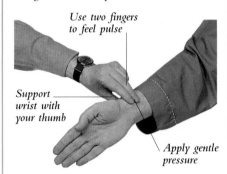

Use two fingers to feel pulse

Support wrist with your thumb

Apply gentle pressure

How to take a pulse Place your fingertips in the hollow just above the wrist creases at the base of the thumb. Count the beats for one minute and record the figure. Try to judge the strength of the pulse as well as the rhythm.

DEALING WITH A HIGH TEMPERATURE

A high temperature (over 102°F/39°C) is usually the result of an infection (*see page 54*), and may be impossible to prevent and difficult to control.

TREATING A HIGH TEMPERATURE
Your aims are to try to lower the temperature and make your relative comfortable. Call the physician if a high temperature persists or you are worried.
Offer the chance to freshen up Ask your relative if he would like to wash, and a change of clothes and sheets.
Monitor room temperature Ensure that the room is adequately ventilated. You can use a fan, but do not overchill.
Provide fluids and food Give him plenty of cold drinks, and offer frequent mouthwashes. Loss of fluid may cause appetite loss and sluggish bowel movements, so provide light meals only.

Offer medication Acetaminophen may lower the temperature. Make sure that you give the correct dosage and check with the pharmacist that it does not conflict with other medication.
Cool with water Sponge your relative all over with tepid water, but do not let him get too cold. Gently dry him afterward. Alternatively, apply a cool compress to his forehead.

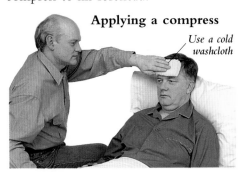

Applying a compress

Use a cold washcloth

DEALING WITH A LOW TEMPERATURE

Hypothermia can occur when the body temperature drops below 95°F (35°C) and if the surrounding temperature is especially cold. Those most at risk are elderly, immobile, and sick people.

TREATING HYPOTHERMIA
Hypothermia is a life-threatening condition, so urgent medical help should always be sought. An elderly person should be rewarmed gradually (*see page 157*). A young, fit person can be rewarmed by having a bath.

PREVENTING HYPOTHERMIA
Take steps to prevent your relative from getting hypothermia.
Regulate room temperature The temperature drops at night, so make sure

that the bedroom is kept at around 64°F (18°C). Seek advice on financial allowances for heating bills for someone with a limited income.
Provide sufficient food and drink Hot food and drink and regular meals are essential. If your relative is immobile, give him a thermos of a hot drink.
Provide effective clothing Several layers of light clothing are more effective than one thick layer. Gloves and socks help keep extremities such as fingers and toes warm. A hat prevents heat loss from the head, especially if someone is bald or has thinning hair.
Encourage movement Exercise helps the circulation of blood. A few minutes walking around the room will help if your relative is able to do so.

BREATHING DIFFICULTIES

IF THE PERSON YOU ARE CARING FOR experiences difficulty breathing, you should seek medical advice immediately. Breathlessness may be a symptom of a short-term illness, such as the flu, but it could also result from a lung condition, such as asthma, or even a heart problem. Treatments range from self-help remedies to the use of specialized equipment.

ALLEVIATING BREATHING DIFFICULTIES

Breathing difficulties can be prevented or minimized by limiting possible environmental factors, and by the person assuming the most comfortable and effective posture to ease breathing.

ENVIRONMENT
A room's atmosphere may aggravate your relative's breathing difficulties. Try to establish whether there are any specific factors that appear to improve or worsen the condition and, if possible, make changes to alleviate the problem.
Ventilate rooms Hot rooms, especially those that are centrally heated, can aggravate respiratory problems. You can help by making sure that:
♦ rooms are adequately ventilated;
♦ the heating is not too high;
♦ the atmosphere is not too dry (a bowl of water placed in the room can increase humidity).
Pinpoint allergies There may be contributing factors to your relative's condition. You can help by:
♦ keeping away known allergens, such as animal fur or feather pillows;
♦ keeping the environment as clean and dust-free as possible.
Encourage outdoor activities Being outside may help alleviate the problem. Encourage your relative to:
♦ go for walks in pollution-free areas;
♦ sit in the garden, if the weather allows.

POSTURE
There are various positions that a person can assume, whether in bed or in a chair, that can make breathing easier. Your relative will probably know which position is most comfortable, so always listen to him. The positions include:
♦ sitting in an upright chair, supported by pillows or a backrest;
♦ sitting upright in a bed with pillows or a specially designed backrest (*see page 87*);
♦ leaning forward with arms supported on a chair or a stool, for temporary relief.

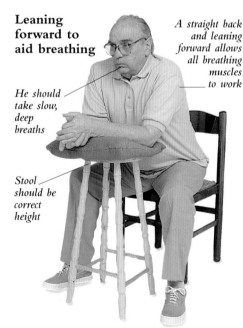

Leaning forward to aid breathing

A straight back and leaning forward allows all breathing muscles to work

He should take slow, deep breaths

Stool should be correct height

MEDICATION FOR BREATHING DIFFICULTIES

Medication can vary from antibiotics for chest infections, to inhalers and oxygen for more long-term breathing difficulties.

PRESCRIBED INHALERS

Someone with a breathing difficulty, such as asthma, will be prescribed an inhaler and shown how to use it; the device enables medication to be inhaled directly into the lungs. Make sure an inhaler and a refill are always readily available. There are different types.

Preventer inhaler A sufferer uses this type of inhaler regularly to prevent an attack.

Reliever inhaler This type of inhaler is used during an attack to open the person's airways quickly.

Spacer This device has a mouthpiece at one end and a hole for the inhaler at the other end. The inhaler is inserted into the spacer and the medication is squirted into it before being breathed in through the mouthpiece. These are often used to enable a child, an elderly person, or someone who is weak to inhale the medication more effectively.

Nebulizer This is a small machine that provides a larger dose of medication than an inhaler. It is only used when breathing difficulties are severe.

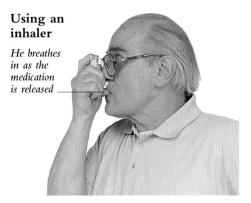

Using an inhaler

He breathes in as the medication is released

RESPIRATORY THERAPY

Breathlessness may be treated with respiratory therapy. Chest respiratory therapy, postural drainage, and breathing techniques are simple treatments that can be carried out at home. In a disorder such as cystic fibrosis, these can help minimize infection by enabling the lungs to stay clear of the sticky mucus brought on by the condition. After surgery, especially when the chest cavity has been opened, breathing exercises can help the person regain normal breathing patterns. Whatever the condition, a respiratory therapist will train you in the techniques that are suitable for your relative's age and condition. Treatment may be required daily, or more often for serious conditions.

STEAM INHALATION

A simple home remedy for loosening phlegm and easing coughing is to add an inhalant to steaming hot water. The person then inhales the steam. Inhalation can be an effective treatment for colds, flu, and mild bronchitis. Ask your pharmacist to recommend an inhalant.

Method Add the inhalant to a bowl of hot water, following the instructions on the bottle, and place it on a table. Ask the person to sit down and place his face over the bowl. Make sure that:
- the water is not *boiling* hot;
- his face is not too close to the water.

Place a towel over his head, large enough to cover his head and the bowl. Advise him to inhale for up to ten minutes and stay with him throughout.

GIVING OXYGEN

Oxygen may be prescribed for chronic chest or heart complaints.

For intermittent use Oxygen is supplied by a cylinder in the home and given via a mask.

For continuous use A machine will be installed in the home. This machine provides a continuous supply of oxygen to the person through nasal tubes.

To aid mobility In addition to a large cylinder, the person may be given a portable cylinder, enabling her to walk around, climb stairs, and leave the house and still receive oxygen.

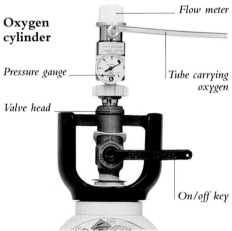

Oxygen cylinder

Flow meter

Pressure gauge

Tube carrying oxygen

Valve head

On/off key

OXYGEN PRECAUTIONS

Always follow instructions carefully:
◆ give oxygen only at the rate prescribed;
◆ monitor oxygen level;
◆ check level of water in any humidifier;
◆ keep cylinders away from fires, open flames, electrical toys, grease, and oil;
◆ do not smoke near oxygen cylinders;
◆ always keep spare supplies;
◆ store cylinders in a cool place.

GIVING OXYGEN BY MASK

1 Before giving oxygen, read the pressure gauge to check how much oxygen the cylinder contains.

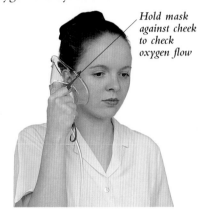

Hold mask against cheek to check oxygen flow

2 Connect the tube of the mask to the cylinder, as instructed. Use the key to open the cylinder valve and adjust the rate of oxygen flow according to the instructions. Check that the oxygen is flowing by holding the mask near your cheek.

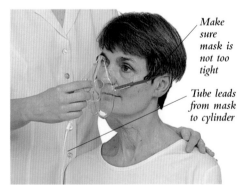

Make sure mask is not too tight

Tube leads from mask to cylinder

3 Arrange the mask over the person's nose and mouth. Record the amount of oxygen given in liters per minute. You may be provided with a mask that delivers a fixed percentage of oxygen.

MEDICATION

THERE ARE TWO CATEGORIES of medication: those that require a doctor's prescription and those that do not. You should have an understanding of why your relative needs to take any medication, and be aware of potential side effects. Your main aims are to make sure medication is taken correctly and, wherever possible, allow your relative to take it by himself.

MEDICATION GUIDELINES

When assisting with medication, follow the basic rules:
◆ check you have the correct medication;
◆ give medication only to the person for whom it has been prescribed;
◆ make sure that the exact quantity prescribed is taken at the recommended times.

PRESCRIBED MEDICATION
Follow the physician's instructions and always read the label and accompanying leaflets. Contact the physician's office or the pharmacist for advice if necessary.

OVER-THE-COUNTER MEDICATION
There has been a huge increase in the availability of over-the-counter drugs, which do not require a prescription. These are available at supermarkets and local stores, as well as at pharmacies. If your relative is already on medication, or if you have any doubts about the drugs you are buying, you should always seek the advice of a pharmacist or physician.

SIDE EFFECTS OF MEDICATION

Read the leaflet supplied with the medication or check with the physician or pharmacist about any side effects.

Drowsiness The person may be advised not to drink alcohol, drive, or operate machinery.

Diet The physician or pharmacist should advise if any dietary restrictions need to be observed.

Adverse reactions Side effects, such as diarrhea, vomiting, dizziness, skin rashes, and any other unexpected problems should be reported to the physician.

DO'S & DON'TS

☑ **Do** wash your hands (*see page 56*) before and after giving medication.

☑ **Do** check the expiration date if the medication has not been used for some time.

☑ **Do** store medication in child-proof containers, especially if they are stored in the refrigerator.

☑ **Do** follow storage instructions.

☑ **Do** dispose of needles and syringes correctly (*see page 58*).

☑ **Do** dispose of unwanted prescription medication.

☒ **Don't** give the medication if it has changed color or has turned cloudy.

☒ **Don't** give the medication if you are unable to read the label.

☒ **Don't** store different pills in one bottle.

☒ **Don't** decant from one bottle into another.

TYPES OF MEDICATION

Liquids Always shake the bottle to mix the constituents thoroughly. Follow the instructions on the bottle and use the correct size of measuring spoon. Don't use the medicine if it has changed color or turned cloudy.

Tablets Some tablets can be crushed and mixed with honey or jam, unless the person has dietary restrictions. Sugar-coated tablets and those that have a shiny shell should be swallowed whole, if possible, with a drink.

Capsules These should not be broken open since they are designed to dissolve slowly in the stomach. They are easier to swallow if placed at the back of the tongue and taken with a drink.

Powders These can be stirred and dissolved in liquids such as water or milk. Mixing them with foods, such as jam or honey, can also make them more palatable, but check that no dietary restrictions apply.

Suppositories and pessaries Suppositories are inserted into the rectum; pessaries into the vagina. The person should insert these according to medical instruction. Do not administer them yourself unless properly instructed.

Creams/lotions Some lotions and creams contain powerful drugs, such as steroids. Always follow the instructions on the tube or bottle. It is advisable to wear latex gloves (*see page 57*) when applying some creams and lotions.

Inhalers These enable a person to inhale drugs to alleviate breathing difficulties (*see page 131*). They may be prescribed with a spacer, to make them easier to use.

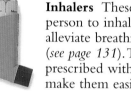

Needles A person who needs regular medication by injection is usually taught how to do this himself. Ensure that the dosage is correct and that needles are disposed of safely (*see page 58*).

MONITORING DOSAGE

The person you are caring for may be on more than one type of medication, and knowing when to take each one can be confusing. To help, a pharmacist can supply the medication in a way that makes it easy to monitor dosage. Normally, he will divide a week's supply into separate daily doses, either in compartmentalized cassettes or blister packs, so that the person can see at a glance which medication to take and

when to take it. Each compartment or pack is labeled with the day and the time the named dose is to be taken.

Advantages This system enables you to:
◆ monitor dosages of medication, while allowing your relative to be independent;
◆ minimize the risk of conflicting medications being taken together;
◆ in an emergency, to know at once which medication the person has taken, so you can report to any medical personnel.

ADMINISTERING EYE, NOSE, AND EAR DROPS

Medications for the eye, nose, and ear usually come in the form of drops. These are sterile and should always be used before the expiration date on the package. If only one eye or ear is affected, make sure that you apply drops to the correct side because it can be dangerous to use medication on healthy organs. When applying eyedrops, do not allow the dropper to come into contact with the eye because this can often spread infection. Wash the dropper if it becomes contaminated. It is common for steroids or drugs such as antibiotics and antihistamines to be given in eyedrop, nose drop, or eardrop form.

APPLYING EYEDROPS

1 Stand behind the person. Ask him to lean his head back against you and look up.

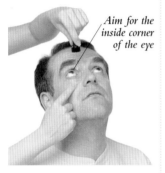

Aim for the inside corner of the eye

2 Give him a tissue to hold against his cheek. Gently pull out the lower eyelid. Squeeze the correct dosage in the space between the lower eyelid and the eyeball, near the inside corner of the eye.

3 The person will automatically close his eye. Ask him to blink a couple of times. This disperses the eyedrop over the whole surface of the eye.

APPLYING NOSE DROPS

1 Ask the person to blow his nose so that any blockage is cleared before applying the drops.

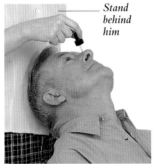

Stand behind him

2 Ask him to tilt his head as far back as possible. Insert the tip of the dropper just inside the nostril and squeeze out the correct dosage. Repeat this procedure for the other nostril.

3 Ask him to sniff to disperse the drops within the nasal cavity. Advise him to stay in the same position for a short while and to refrain from blowing his nose for at least 20 minutes.

APPLYING EARDROPS

1 Ask the person to tilt her head so that the affected ear is uppermost.

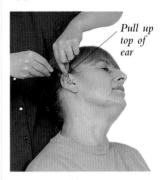

Pull up top of ear

2 Hold the top of the ear. Position the dropper just above the opening. Allow drops to trickle into the ear canal.

3 Ask the person to keep her head still, in the same position, for a few minutes.

4 Place a piece of cotton just over the opening to the ear. Under no circumstances should the cotton be pushed into the ear canal.

WOUND CARE

A WOUND IS A BREAK IN THE SKIN, and may be the result of an injury, a disease, or an operation. The kind of care needed depends on the size and severity of the wound. If the wound is large and gaping, you should seek professional help. Wounds caused by an operation, or conditions such as varicose ulcers, may require regular aftercare, and this will usually be carried out by a nurse.

THE HEALING PROCESS

When any part of the body has been damaged, as a result of, for example, a cut, wound, or pressure sore, tissues adjacent to the injured area will begin to repair the damage. If tissue has been lost, as occurs with a burn or an abscess, or if the affected area has been contaminated in any way, it will take longer for the body to heal itself.

The body repairs the damaged area in the following way:

◆ The wound bleeds and the ruptured area is filled with blood that clots quickly, then dries to form a scab.

◆ White blood cells begin to destroy and remove dead and damaged tissue.

◆ Cells grow rapidly in the clotted blood.

◆ Firm, fibrous tissues form across the wound and may become a scar.

TREATING A WOUND

As a caregiver, you may be asked to help the registered nurse to dress a wound or have to deal with a wound in an emergency. It is a good idea to keep sterile dressings (*see page 162*) in your basic first-aid kit at home. Your main aims when dressing a wound are:

◆ to prevent bacteria from entering the wound;
◆ to hasten healing and alleviate pain.

PREVENTING INFECTION

To keep the wound from becoming infected, always:
◆ wash your hands before treatment (*see page 56*);
◆ wear sterile latex gloves, if possible (*see page 57*);
◆ clean the area so that dirt is washed away;
◆ cover the wound with a dressing, preferably sterile;
◆ dry the surrounding skin with a clean towel;
◆ secure dressings properly and keep them dry;
◆ dispose of used dressings and gloves (*see page 58*).

An infected wound Seek medical advice if the wound begins to ooze, the skin around the wound becomes red, there is swelling or discomfort, or the person complains of feeling hot or being in pain.

AIDING THE HEALING PROCESS

Babies and children heal much more rapidly than someone who is sick or elderly. Those who have an underlying condition that requires medicines such as steroids, or others that suppress their immunity, may heal less quickly.

What the body requires In order for a wound to heal, a person needs to be physically healthy. If a wound fails to heal, it may be because of an underlying condition, such as anemia, so you should seek the advice of a healthcare professional, such as a physician or registered nurse.

CHAPTER 13

PALLIATIVE CARE

The aim of palliative care is to ensure that a person
who has a seemingly incurable condition suffers as little as
possible, and that all her physical, psychological, and spiritual needs
are satisfied. The emphasis is on relieving and easing each
symptom of the illness, rather than curing the disease itself, and
on facilitating a peaceful and dignified death.
Palliative care is not necessarily short-term – where
the disease is degenerative, care may stretch over many years.
Many people prefer to die at home in familiar surroundings and
in the company of their families; this is usually feasible only
if specialist help is provided by a physician or registered nurse,
with adequate support from a hospice or other
appropriate healthcare professionals.

CLOSE RELATIONSHIPS

Although caring for someone who is dying is
stressful and upsetting, it can give people the chance to say
goodbye properly. It may also reunite a family, forge friendships,
and provide an opportunity to express affection. Close
relationships between the caregiver, the family, and friends
are likely to continue after the death, and can be
a great source of comfort and support
to those who are grieving.

FACING DEATH

FINDING OUT THAT SOMEONE is going to die brings with it a wide range of emotions. Your dying relative may fear death, pain, or simply the unknown. You may have fears about seeing someone who is close to you suffer, and you may worry about being left alone once she has died. These fears are completely understandable; talking about them openly may help you begin to cope.

DO'S & DON'TS

The quality of care you provide will improve if you also look after your own needs.

☑ **Do** acknowledge your own grief. It is a sign of human strength, not human failing.

☑ **Do** turn to healthcare professionals for their support, and take advantage of their experience and expertise.

☑ **Do** seek the help of volunteer caregivers.

☒ **Don't** feel guilty if you are angry or frightened that your relative is dying. These emotions are natural, but try to confide in others rather than depress your relative.

☒ **Don't** bottle up your emotions, since this may create even more stress.

☒ **Don't** regard yourself as useless. You are providing essential support in a difficult time of need.

WHEN THE NEWS IS BROKEN

You may be one of the first people to be informed that your relative is terminally ill, but it is the responsibility of the healthcare professional, not you, to inform her of this. You will, however, need to be prepared for how you handle this delicate subject.

Be informed If possible, try to be present when your relative receives the news: by listening and learning about her condition you may be able to provide comfort and support later.

Be honest If your relative asks you to expand on any detail, try to tell the truth as sensitively as possible. If there are any questions you cannot answer, seek the advice of a healthcare professional.

Be discreet Your relative may not wish to discuss death, or may even refuse to believe she is dying. If you need to talk, discuss the issue with other family members or with an outsider, such as the physician.

THE IMPORTANCE OF COMMUNICATION

As death approaches, it is important that the dying person is encouraged to share her feelings.

Talking Do not be put off if she is unable to speak; listening to you talking can be very soothing.

Listening If she is able to express her wishes and sentiments, listen patiently and carefully; this is one of the most important things you can do for her.

Writing If she finds it difficult to talk, suggest that she writes down her feelings.

Touching Hold her hand; this can soothe anxieties and communicate reassurance and affection.

Counseling Your relative may benefit from talking to someone outside her family and close friends, such as a professional counselor (*see page 22*).

STAGES OF GRIEF

After the initial shock of learning that someone is terminally ill, there are various emotions and stages of grief that may affect those concerned. It can be an unsettling time; one moment you may be deeply emotional, the next you may feel numb. You will be able to cope better, and support your relative more effectively, if you are as open as possible about your feelings.

DEALING WITH GRIEF

EMOTION	HOW IT IS EXPRESSED	HOW TO DEAL WITH IT
Denial	◆ Your dying relative may reject the diagnosis, even after many doctors have been consulted. Be prepared to acknowledge that she may never accept the reality. ◆ It is often easier to ignore the implications of death than to face up to the reality of it. Some people may conceal shock and try to cope by behaving as if nothing has happened.	◆ You should listen patiently and sensitively to your relative. If she does not acknowledge that she is dying, do not press the point; she will deal with it in her own way. ◆ Discuss your feelings, if possible, with your dying relative and close family and friends. If everyone is able to accept the reality, this could reduce the emotional stress that is felt later.
Anger	◆ The dying person is likely to feel angry because she is afraid of death. She may direct her anger at you and others who care for her, which may be difficult to handle. She may also become irritable and depressed. ◆ You and others who are close to your relative may feel angry that she is dying.	◆ Accept that anger is a natural step toward your relative accepting her death, and try not to take personally any anger that is directed at you. ◆ Anger can be a good way for both of you to vent your feelings. Ask healthcare professionals for advice on how best to deal with angry confrontations.
Acceptance	◆ Having worked through denial and anger, your relative may finally accept that she is dying. ◆ She may ask for your help with practical arrangements, such as making a will. ◆ She may feel ready to have visitors and make the most of the time she has left.	◆ Offer to help your relative put her affairs in order. Reassure her that you will try to simplify issues and take responsibility for what has to be done. ◆ Encourage visitors to come at a time when your relative is feeling at her best, so that she does not become agitated or exhausted.

PRACTICAL CARE

WHEN YOU ARE CARING for a dying relative, one of your main aims will be to give her the best quality of life possible. This means making sure that she is comfortable, free of pain, and, to alleviate boredom and depression, has enough to keep her occupied. Always try to respect your relative's wishes and encourage her to be as independent as possible.

PROFESSIONAL SUPPORT

You may feel unable to give your relative enough time, offer adequate care, or cope with the many demands without help. In this situation, you may need to seek part- or full-time professional help. Consult your relative's physician for advice and information on what help is available.

Think ahead Anticipate when you might need the extra help and try to make the necessary arrangements before you find yourself in a crisis situation.

Seek short-term help Some local agencies and charities have units that provide short-term care.

Seek full-time help Hospices, nursing homes, or specialist organizations (*see pages 174–76*) provide care for those who are terminally ill, and help and advise the caregivers who look after the person.

COMFORTABLE SURROUNDINGS

If your relative is confined to bed or to the house, personal space will be extremely important to her. You can help by trying to make her feel comfortable and in control of her surroundings.

THE ROOM

For your relative's comfort, make sure her surroundings are kept clean and pleasant.
Ventilate the room A stuffy room can be unpleasant: open the windows but avoid creating a draft.
Find the right level of light Arrange the curtains so that as much – or as little – light comes into the room to suit your relative's needs.
Make the room look pleasant Fresh flowers will add color and fragrance, and liven up the room. Potpourri and scented candles may freshen the air.

VISITORS

Before encouraging friends or relatives to visit, make sure your relative wants to see them. Ideally, visits should be restricted to people with whom your relative feels comfortable. Do not be afraid to cancel visits if you feel that she is unable to cope. Remember, also, that too many visitors may put a strain on you as the caregiver.
Monitor the length of visits Short, frequent visits are better than irregular, drawn-out ones that may be exhausting for your relative.
Restrict the number of visitors One or two visitors at a time are less overwhelming than large groups.
Prepare visitors Try to prepare visitors for your relative's appearance and attitude. They may find it awkward or feel shocked or upset if she is physically different or very depressed.

DAILY CARE

Encourage your relative to eat and drink, keep clean, and generally look after herself. Accept, however, that she may not want to do so. Inform the physician if your relative has any uncomfortable symptoms, such as bowel problems, vomiting, or pressure sores.

EATING AND DRINKING

Eating meals She may prefer small, appetizing snacks at frequent intervals rather than three large meals a day. Make a note of any changes in appetite, and report them to the healthcare professional.

Drinking fluids Even if your relative does not wish to eat, encourage her to drink plenty of fluids.

Indulgences Allow your relative to have alcohol or cigarettes if she requests them.

PERSONAL HYGIENE AND APPEARANCE

Washing Encourage your relative to wash and bathe for her personal comfort and dignity. If she is confined to bed, you may be shown how to give her a bedbath (*see page 99*).

Personal grooming You can help by offering to wash and brush your relative's hair and cut her fingernails and toenails. A man may feel better if he has had a shave, and a woman may require assistance with applying makeup (*see page 101*), especially when visitors are expected.

Getting dressed Unless your relative is confined to bed, it is not necessary for her to stay in sleepwear. Encourage her to get dressed because this can give her dignity and bolster confidence.

Using the toilet Encourage your relative to get out of bed to use the toilet. If she cannot, obtain toilet aids that allow maximum independence (*see page 114*).

LIVING LIFE TO THE FULL

Mobility If your relative is able, she should be encouraged to be mobile, even if this only means getting out of bed to sit in a chair.

Hobbies If she is physically able, try to stimulate interest in pastimes that you know she enjoys. This may give her pleasure, and the encouragement she needs to live the remainder of her life to the full.

HELPING TO MINIMIZE PAIN

A dying person's greatest fear may be the prospect of coping with pain.

Reassure your relative You can reassure your relative that from the time of diagnosis, and throughout her care, she will be given medicines to minimize pain.

Act promptly Should she suffer pain at any time, inform a healthcare professional so that the situation can be rectified as soon as possible.

Find out about specialized equipment The use of specialized equipment will be explained to you, and administered under the supervision of a healthcare professional. For example, a pain-relieving device such as a TENS (Transcutaneous Electric Nerve Stimulator) may be suggested, or syringe pumps to administer pain-relieving medicines. Speak to the physician about what is suitable.

Consider alternative therapies Your relative may prefer to try techniques such as reflexology, aromatherapy, and visualization.

TOWARD THE END OF LIFE

AS THE HEALTH OF YOUR RELATIVE DETERIORATES, you may notice signs that indicate she is dying. As life recedes, she will become weaker and sleep more frequently and for longer periods. In some cases, death may occur without warning. Your main – although perhaps daunting – aim is to make your relative's last days as peaceful and as pain-free as possible.

PLANNING AHEAD

If your relative has expressed any wishes before she dies, these should be honored.

Living will A living will (*Advance Directive*) allows a person to refuse or express a choice on future treatment should she become too ill to do so later. Medical staff are usually sympathetic to living wills. To avoid complications at a later stage, make sure that the documents required by each state in which she lives have been properly filled out and notarized; states vary in their regulations. Inform family members of her wishes in case they try to intervene at a later stage. Legally, relatives have little power to change any decision that has been made.

Donor card If your relative carries a donor card, find out what her exact intentions are concerning donation.

MAKING SOMEONE COMFORTABLE

Dying is often a slow, peaceful process. Your relative may slip in and out of consciousness, or perhaps lose consciousness altogether.

Talk and hold hands Even if your relative is unconscious, she may still be able to hear and feel. Do not be afraid to talk to her or hold her hand because this can provide comfort.

Maintain privacy Be guided by your relative's wishes and general condition.

Arrange spiritual support A visit from a spiritual adviser, such as a priest, could help give your relative the strength and courage to face death.

MAKING ARRANGEMENTS IN ADVANCE

One of the most delicate areas you may have to discuss with your relative is her funeral, but do not force the issue. If she wants to talk about it, ask if she has any preferences regarding the following:

◆ whether she wishes to be buried or cremated;
◆ the type of service: any hymns, music, or readings;
◆ the type of headstone or memorial, and inscription;
◆ where the ashes should be scattered.

FIND OUT IMPORTANT INFORMATION

Find out the names, addresses, and telephone numbers of people who should be notified of death and locate the following documents:

◆ the will
◆ medical insurance card
◆ Social Security card
◆ birth and marriage certificates
◆ insurance, pension, and other policies
◆ bank details

THE ROLE OF THE VOLUNTEER

THE DEMANDS ON YOU if you are a volunteer caregiver outside the family circle will be great at this time. Family members and friends of the person dying may need you as much as, if not more than, the person in your care, and this can be particularly stressful. To help you cope with the demands and strains of your role, bear in mind what people will expect of you during this time.

COMPLEMENTARY CARE

Your responsibility as a caregiver outside the family circle is to complement, not dominate, the care regime. Try to achieve a balance between supporting the needs of the dying person and those who are close to her. Allow family and friends to be involved in her care.

ESSENTIAL QUALITIES OF THE CAREGIVER

As a volunteer, you must be a source of strength and support at all times; not only to the person in your care, but also to her close family and friends.

Sensitivity and tact You will need these skills as you support the home caregiver, the person who is dying, and her relatives. Try not to intrude into their grief, and allow the home caregiver to do as much or as little of the caring as she wishes. Your role is to offer only the practical and psychological help that might be required of you. Allow friends and family as much privacy as you can. Respect their wishes at all times, particularly those who are religiously or spiritually motivated.

Sympathy and patience Be as sympathetic and patient as you can. Listen to the dying person's friends and relatives if they want to talk about their feelings; leave them alone if they do not. Try to be patient when people repeat themselves, and show them that you are aware of their needs. If a person refuses to acknowledge what is happening, you should respect this.

Calmness and composure It is natural for grieving relatives to feel increasingly emotional and concerned as the dying person becomes weaker. You will need to remain calm at all times, particularly in the immediate period after the person has died, in order to provide comfort, reassurance, and support.

SPIRITUAL AND CULTURAL NEEDS

You may be well aware of the dying person's spiritual views but, if not, you may find it useful to acquaint yourself with her beliefs and customs.

Obtain information Ask the person, or her family and close friends, about her beliefs. Obtain additional information if needed (*see page 37*).

Find out about religious customs Consult the spiritual adviser, if there is one, so that you are aware of any particular customs.

Show respect Once you are familiar with the person's spiritual needs, try to bear them in mind at all times.

Arrange special visits To gain the courage to face death, the person may ask you to arrange a visit from a member of her religious community, such as a priest.

When Death Occurs

Y OU CAN NEVER REALLY PREPARE yourself fully for the moment of your relative's death. The experience will be different for everyone, and each person will have different ways of reacting to it. Being present when someone dies is an ultimately personal, intimate, and even positive experience that is intrinsically bound up with your relationship with that person.

CASE STUDY

NAME: JANINE
AGE: 40

J anine had cared for her mother, Valerie, who had Alzheimer's disease, for more than five years. She had even moved into Valerie's house when her mother could no longer look after herself. Although Janine had often thought about her mother's death, she was not prepared for it to happen suddenly.

One day, Janine found Valerie slumped on the sofa. She checked for signs of life and called her mother's physician, who later confirmed that Valerie had suffered a cardiac arrest minutes before Janine had entered the room.

As she came to terms with her mother's death, Janine realized how shocked she had been by the suddenness of it, but thinking back, she was glad that they had had so much time together before she died.

IF SOMEONE DIES AT HOME

Although death may sometimes be sudden and unexpected, it is in many instances a gentle slipping away rather than a dramatic event. Try to prepare yourself as much as possible and know what to do if your relative dies at home.

HOW DO I KNOW IF SOMEONE HAS DIED?

If you are not sure whether your relative has actually passed away, the following simple checks may be useful indicators:
♦ check the pulse (*see page 128*) and look, listen, and feel carefully for any signs of breathing;
♦ check the eyes, looking for signs of movement. Recheck these signs after a few minutes.

WHAT DO I DO WHEN SOMEONE HAS DIED?

Before you do anything, make sure you observe any religious customs. Inform the physician and the family and, if you feel comfortable dealing with the body and any equipment, follow the procedures below.
Call the physician When he arrives, tell him the approximate time and nature of the death so that he can produce a death certificate (*see opposite*).
Inform the family Close members of the family may wish to spend some time alone with the person before the undertaker removes the body.
Lay the body flat Remove the pillows from the bed, straighten the body, and lay it flat.
Switch off equipment If there is any electrical equipment in place, turn it off. You do not need to detach any equipment from the body.
Call the undertaker The undertaker will remove any syringes or catheters and take the body to the mortuary, where it will remain until the funeral.

FINAL ARRANGEMENTS

AFTER THE DEATH, everyone involved will experience a range of emotions as they begin to come to terms with what has happened. Accept any offers of help to make funeral and other arrangements. You may feel detached as you organize the funeral and deal with formalities; it is very normal to feel this way and for the reality of the death not to sink in until later.

ARRANGEMENTS AFTER DEATH

There are various documents you will need to obtain following the person's death:
- a signed death certificate from the physician;
- the relevant details and documents for registering the death (*see right*).

With these documents you can get a death certificate from your local registry office for which there is a fee. You will need at least three copies of the death certificate for legal, insurance, and banking purposes. Contact the Social Security Administration and other relevant agencies to cancel any benefit payments.

ARRANGING THE FUNERAL

If you discussed the funeral with your relative before she died, you may already know what kind of service is required. The funeral director will:
- contact the place of burial or cremation;
- discuss the type of service you require;
- arrange a suitable date and time for the service.

You will need to:
- notify friends and relatives of the date and location;
- organize flowers, if required, for the service;
- organize a location for a post-funeral gathering.

TALKING TO OTHER MOURNERS

For some, the loss of a loved one may become real for the first time at the funeral.

Acknowledge the loss Talking about your relative and sharing memories with others who knew her will help the grieving process.

Celebrate life The funeral need not be a sad and solemn affair. With the help of those people who mattered most to your relative you can make it a time to celebrate the importance of her life.

REGISTERING A DEATH

Obtain a list of deadlines from the probate clerk in your relative's town. If your relative had property in more than one place, you must contact the probate clerk in each town. Provide the clerk with the following information and documentation:
- certificate of the cause of death (from the health department or funeral director);
- full name (and maiden name, if relevant) and address of deceased;
- birth certificate of the deceased;
- deceased's last full-time occupation, even if she was retired;
- the name and occupation of spouse, if relevant;
- marital status of the deceased and date of birth of surviving spouse;
- insurance number, pension, and benefit details of the deceased.

AFTER DEATH

THE WEEKS THAT FOLLOW the death may prove to be difficult for you as you adjust from being a full-time caregiver. With less to occupy you, it is easy to dwell on your loss rather than look forward to the future. Now is the time for you to enjoy the company of people who care about you and those who miss your relative, and give and receive sympathy and support.

CASE STUDY

NAME: ELIZABETH
AGE: 56

Elizabeth had been her husband's caregiver for two years, and she was devastated when he died. For a few weeks, she felt uneasy about leaving the house, even to go shopping, but she knew she had to get on with her life.

Then, one day, she saw an advertisement for an evening course in pottery. Taking her courage in her hands, Elizabeth enrolled on the course. On the first evening, she discovered she had no real talent for pottery, but she did meet Daphne, also recently widowed. The two women soon developed a close friendship fueled by many shared interests.

Of course Elizabeth still missed her husband and thought of him often, yet by making a determined effort she was able to maintain a fulfilling life.

GRIEVING

While you may have anticipated the grief you would feel after losing a loved one, you may have grown accustomed to suppressing your feelings in the interests of caring for the person. Although it may be difficult, the ability to express your grief is an essential part of the recovery procedure. There are many ways you can help yourself through the grieving process.

Be patient Allow yourself the time to grieve.

Be open Try not to suppress your emotions. It is far healthier to shed tears and express your grief to others.

Be honest Do not feel guilty about being relieved or angry that your relative has died; these reactions often follow the loss of someone close, particularly if the person suffered, or you cared for her for a long time.

Be positive Try not to dwell solely on feelings of loss; try to use your grief positively by expressing the joy of having known your relative.

Be resourceful There are many organizations that provide advice and counseling (*see pages 174–76*); most hospices provide bereavement counseling.

GIVING AND RECEIVING SUPPORT

Grieving is a long process and it is important that support is maintained throughout this period. Sharing and exchanging sympathy can be a great comfort and will help all concerned to grieve.

Express yourself Try to express how you feel and how you intend to cope without the person.

Reminisce Be open: others may wish to talk to you about your relative and reminisce about the past.

Be sociable Make the effort to see people. If possible, try to maintain contact with those who have helped you; their continuing support may help you adjust to your new circumstances.

CHAPTER 14

EMERGENCY CARE

As a caregiver you need to know what emergency
action to take if your relative is seriously ill or injured.
The following section is not a substitute for first-aid training,
which is a practical skill, but if you familiarize yourself with
the techniques shown, it will help you administer fast and
effective treatments for potentially life-threatening conditions.
Remember, you can only do what you believe to be correct: some
conditions inevitably lead to death, even in the best medical
hands. Courses in first aid and cardiopulmonary resuscitation are
offered by local branches of the American Red Cross and the
American Heart Association (*see page 174*).

CONTENTS

WHAT TO DO IN AN EMERGENCY

WHEN TO CALL AN AMBULANCE

◆ IF YOU HAVE A HELPER, always send him to call an ambulance immediately.

◆ IF YOU ARE ALONE AND VICTIM IS NOT BREATHING due to injury or drowning, resuscitate for one minute before calling an ambulance. For any other adult victim, call an ambulance as soon as you have discovered that breathing is absent, then continue to resuscitate the victim until help arrives.

◆ IF YOU ARE ALONE AND AN UNCONSCIOUS VICTIM IS BREATHING, place him in the recovery position before you leave him to call an ambulance.

1 ASSESS THE VICTIM (*see opposite*)

If he is conscious	If he is unconscious

Treat any injuries (*see pages 153–60*).	Go to step 2.

2 OPEN AIRWAY AND CHECK BREATHING (*see opposite*)

If he is breathing	If he is not breathing

Place him in the recovery position (*see page 150*).	Go to step 3.

3 GIVE RESCUE BREATHING (*see page 151*)

Go to step 4.

4 CHECK THE PULSE (*see page 151*)

If pulse is present	If pulse is absent

Continue rescue breathing and keep checking the pulse.	Go to step 5.

5 GIVE CPR (*see page 152*)

Give a combination of chest compressions and rescue breathing until help arrives.

UNCONSCIOUSNESS

I F A PERSON COLLAPSES in front of you, immediately establish whether or not he is conscious. If he is unconscious, you must open his airway, check whether or not he is breathing and, if necessary, begin resuscitation. For information on when to call an ambulance, see the chart opposite.

ASSESSING THE VICTIM

1 CHECK FOR CONSCIOUSNESS Ask the victim a question and gently shake his shoulders. If there is no response, the victim is unconscious.

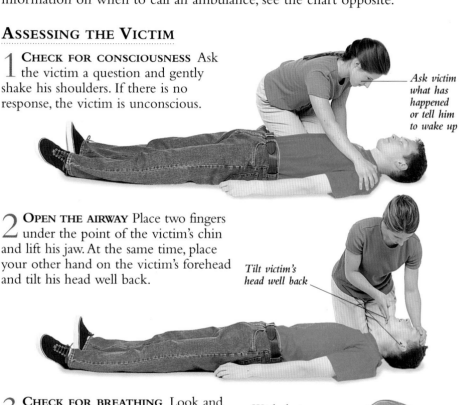

Ask victim what has happened or tell him to wake up

2 OPEN THE AIRWAY Place two fingers under the point of the victim's chin and lift his jaw. At the same time, place your other hand on the victim's forehead and tilt his head well back.

Tilt victim's head well back

3 CHECK FOR BREATHING Look and listen for breathing and feel for breath on your cheek for at least 5 seconds.

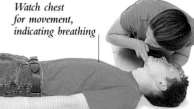

Watch chest for movement, indicating breathing

IF BREATHING IS PRESENT, place in the recovery position, *see page 150* ▶

IF BREATHING IS ABSENT, give rescue breathing, *see page 151* ▶

IF BREATHING IS PRESENT

IF THE VICTIM IS BREATHING and you need to leave him alone to call an ambulance, place him in the recovery position to keep his tongue from blocking his throat and to prevent him from inhaling vomit. If you suspect spinal injury, however, the victim should not be moved.

RECOVERY POSITION

1 **POSITION HAND** Tuck the hand nearest to you, arm straight and palm uppermost, under the victim's thigh.

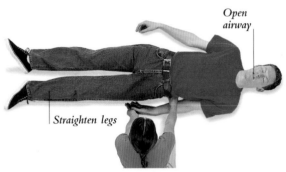

Open airway

Straighten legs

> **IF** you suspect spinal injury do not turn the victim; this could cause paralysis.

2 **PREPARE TO ROLL VICTIM** Bring the arm farthest from you across the victim's chest. Place his hand, palm outward, against his cheek. With your other hand, pull up the knee farthest from you.

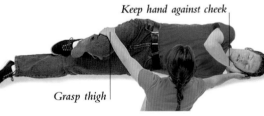

Keep hand against cheek

Grasp thigh

3 **ROLL VICTIM TOWARD YOU** Keeping his hand pressed against his cheek, pull at his thigh and roll him onto his side. Use your knees to support him and prevent him from rolling forward.

4 **MAKE ANY NECESSARY ADJUSTMENTS** Check the position of the victim: his head should be tilted back; his hip and knee should be at right angles to his body; his lower arm should be free and lying along his back.

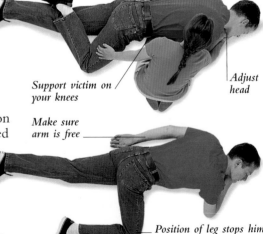

Support victim on your knees

Adjust head

Make sure arm is free

☎ Call an ambulance. Record breathing and pulse rate (*see page 161*).

Position of leg stops him from rolling forward

IF BREATHING IS ABSENT

I F A VICTIM IS NOT BREATHING, you must give rescue breathing. The most common form is mouth-to-mouth, but for a person who has had his voice box removed use the mouth-to-stoma technique (*see box below*).

RESCUE BREATHING

1 **REMOVE ANY OBSTRUCTION** Look into the victim's mouth and remove any *obvious* obstruction.

2 **MAINTAIN OPEN AIRWAY** Keep two fingers under his chin and the other on his forehead, to tilt his head back.

3 **PINCH THE NOSE** Using your index finger and thumb of the hand that is resting on his forehead, pinch his nostrils tightly closed to prevent air escaping.

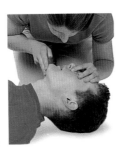

4 **BLOW INTO THE MOUTH** Take a full breath. Place your lips around the victim's mouth. Make a good seal and blow into his mouth until the chest rises. Take two seconds for full inflation. Remove your lips, allow the chest to fall fully, and repeat once.

MOUTH-TO-STOMA BREATHING

If a person's voice box (*larynx*) has been removed, rescue breaths must be given through the opening in the front of the neck (*stoma*). If he is a "partial neck breather," cover the mouth and nose with your fingers to keep air from escaping.

AFTER GIVING TWO RESCUE BREATHS, assess for circulation **see below** ▼

ASSESSING FOR CIRCULATION

C HECK THE PULSE. Use two fingers to feel for the pulse on the side of the neck. While you are doing this, look for any signs of recovery, such as return of color to the skin and any movement.

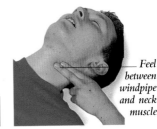

Feel between windpipe and neck muscle

CHECK the pulse for 5–10 seconds.

IF CIRCULATION IS PRESENT, continue rescue breathing **see above** ▶

IF CIRCULATION IS ABSENT, give cardiopulmonary resuscitation **see p.152** ▶

IF CIRCULATION IS PRESENT

IF THE PULSE IS PRESENT, continue rescue breathing. Check the pulse again and look for signs of recovery (*see page 151*) after every 12 breaths or one minute. If at any time the pulse is absent, begin cardiopulmonary resuscitation immediately (*see below*).

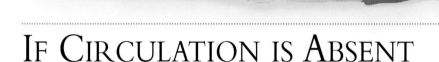

IF CIRCULATION IS ABSENT

IF THERE IS NO PULSE or sign of recovery, you will have to provide an artificial circulation by giving cardiopulmonary resuscitation (CPR). This is a combination of chest compressions and rescue breathing.

GIVING CPR

1 **POSITION YOUR FINGERS** Place the middle finger of your lower hand where the ribs meet the breastbone, and your index finger on the breastbone.

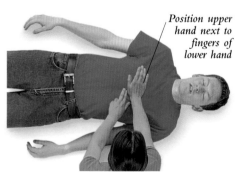

Position upper hand next to fingers of lower hand

2 **POSITION OTHER HAND** Place the heel of your other hand on the breastbone. Slide it down to your index finger and intertwine your fingers.

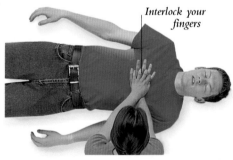

Interlock your fingers

3 **BEGIN CHEST COMPRESSIONS** Lean well over the victim with your arms straight. Press down on the breastbone to depress it approximately 1½–2in (4–5cm). Complete 15 chest compressions, aiming for a rate of about 100 per minute.

4 **GIVE TWO RESCUE BREATHS** (*see page 151*) Continue alternating 15 compressions with 2 rescue breaths until help arrives.

HEART ATTACK

A HEART ATTACK most commonly occurs when the blood supply to part of the heart muscle is obstructed, for example, by a clot in one of the coronary arteries. Angina can be the body's way of warning of a heart attack, so medical help should be sought immediately. This condition occurs when narrowed arteries cannot deliver enough blood to meet the demands of exertion or excitement.

RECOGNITION
There may be:
◆ vicelike chest pain, starting at mid-chest and possibly radiating to the neck and the left arm
◆ breathlessness and discomfort in the upper abdomen
◆ sudden faintness or giddiness
◆ ashen skin and blue lips
◆ a rapid pulse, becoming weaker
◆ collapse

WHAT YOU SHOULD DO

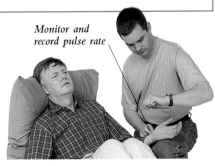

Monitor and record pulse rate

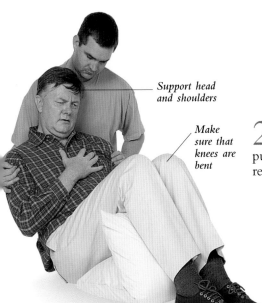

Support head and shoulders

Make sure that knees are bent

2 **MONITOR THE VICTIM** Check and record the victim's breathing and pulse rate (*see page 161*). Be prepared to resuscitate (*see pages 151–52*).

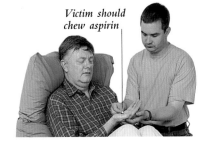

Victim should chew aspirin

1 **MAKE THE VICTIM COMFORTABLE** A half-sitting position with knees bent is usually best.

☎ **Call an ambulance.** Tell the dispatcher you suspect a heart attack.

3 **GIVE THE VICTIM ONE ASPIRIN** Tell him to chew, not swallow whole.

DO NOT give him any water.

CHOKING

IF A PERSON SWALLOWS FOOD that has been inadequately chewed and hurriedly swallowed, she may choke. This can block the throat or induce muscle spasms. Prompt action is required, and you should be prepared to resuscitate (*see pages 151–52*).

> ### RECOGNITION
> There will be:
> ◆ difficulty speaking and breathing;
> ◆ initially, a congested face, and later, gray-blue skin;
> ◆ signs of distress, such as grasping the neck.

WHAT YOU SHOULD DO

> **IF** the victim becomes unconscious ☎ **call an ambulance.** Then, give two rescue breaths; if they do not go in, sweep her mouth with your finger; then give abdominal thrusts.

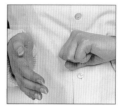

1 **POSITION HAND** Make a fist and position your hand with the thumb side against the victim's abdomen.

2 **GIVE ABDOMINAL THRUSTS** Grasp your fist with your other hand. Pull sharply inward and upward.

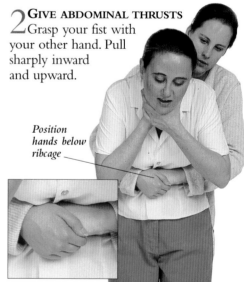

Position hands below ribcage

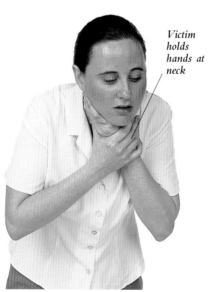

Victim holds hands at neck

HOW TO RECOGNIZE CHOKING A choking victim may hold her hands to her neck, or make very high-pitched, squeaky sounds. Ask if she can breathe.

3 **CONTINUE THRUSTS** until the obstruction clears and the victim can cough or breathe; she becomes unconscious; or medical help arrives.

BURNS

WHEN TREATING BURNS that are deep or those that extend over a large area, you must act quickly to cool the burn, relieve pain, and minimize the extent of the injury. You must also prevent infection, check the victim's breathing, and be prepared to resuscitate her (*see pages 151–52*). Treatment of common, superficial burns is shown below.

> **DO NOT** remove any clothing or material that is sticking to the burned area.
>
> **DO NOT** apply any lotions, ointments, or fat.
>
> **DO NOT** touch the burned area or burst any blisters.
>
> **DO NOT** cover a facial burn.

WHAT YOU SHOULD DO

Cool burn for 2–3 minutes in cold water

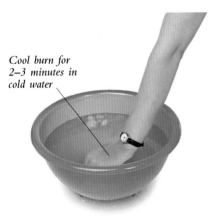

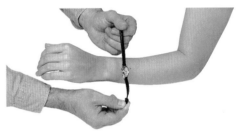

1 SUBMERGE IN COLD WATER Thorough cooling of the burn, by plunging the affected area into a bowl of cold water or ice, may take 2–3 minutes, but this must not delay removal of the victim to the hospital if there is a medical emergency.

2 MONITOR BREATHING Watch for any signs that the victim is having difficulty breathing while you cool the burn, and be prepared to resuscitate (*see pages 151–52*) if necessary.

3 REMOVE CLOTHING AND JEWELRY Remove these if they are on or around the burned area.

4 COVER THE WOUND Use a sterile dressing to protect against infection.

5 MONITOR THE VICTIM Stay with the victim and treat her for shock (*see page 160*), if necessary.

> More severe burns require different first aid. If the burned area has a white or charred appearance, cool the burn by pouring large amounts of cold water on it. Cover the burned area with thick, sterile, dry dressing or clean cloth. ☎ **Call an ambulance.** Give the dispatcher details of the injury.

SEVERE BLEEDING

SPURTING BLOOD, or severe bleeding that does not stop within five minutes, can be life-threatening. You must take action to stop the bleeding immediately. Be prepared to resuscitate the victim if she loses consciousness (*see pages 151–52*) and treat her for shock (*see page 160*) if necessary.

(*see pages 151–52*) ... (*see page 160*)

PROTECTING YOURSELF

If possible, use disposable latex gloves (*see page 57*) and wash your hands well in soap and water, before and after treatment. If you have any sores, cuts, or open wounds, cover them with a waterproof adhesive dressing to prevent any cross-infection.

WHAT YOU SHOULD DO

1 **EXPOSE WOUND** Wearing gloves, if a pair is available, remove or cut clothing from the injured area.

2 **APPLY DIRECT PRESSURE** Preferably using a clean pad or sterile dressing, press the wound for 10 minutes to give the blood time to clot.

3 **RAISE THE INJURED LIMB** Support it above the level of the victim's heart.

4 **LAY VICTIM DOWN** This will reduce the blood flow to the site of the injury and minimize the chance of shock

Keep limb raised

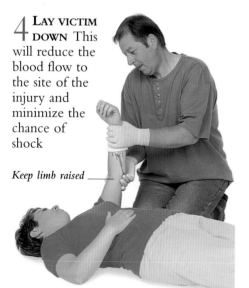

5 **APPLY A DRESSING OR BANDAGE** Leave any original pad in place. If any blood seeps through, apply an additional dressing.

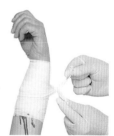

DO NOT bandage too tightly.

IF there is an object protruding from the wound, build up padding on either side of it, until you can bandage over it without applying any pressure.

☎ **Call an ambulance.** Explain the severity of the injury to the dispatcher.

6 **MONITOR VICTIM** Check and record breathing, pulse rate, and level of response (*see page 161*). Treat for shock (*see page 160*), if necessary.

HYPOTHERMIA

PEOPLE WHO ARE immobile, frail, or sick (particularly the elderly) are susceptible to hypothermia. This condition develops when the body temperature falls below 95°F (35°C). An elderly person's body loses its sensitivity to cold so she may not be aware of a drop in her body temperature. Lack of agility, chronic illness, and fatigue can all increase the risk of hypothermia, as can a poorly heated home. If the correct preventive measures are taken (*see page 129*), there is no reason why indoor hypothermia should occur.

RECOGNITION
There may be: ◆ temperature of below 95°F (35°C) ◆ slow, weakening pulse ◆ shivering, and cold, pale, dry skin ◆ lethargy ◆ slow, shallow breathing ◆ apathy, disorientation, irrational behavior.

WHAT YOU SHOULD DO

1 REWARM GRADUALLY Cover an elderly victim with layers of blankets in a room temperature of approximately 77°F (25°C).

> **DO NOT** give the victim any alcohol.

> **DO NOT** allow an elderly person to have a bath or use direct heat sources, such as hot-water bottles or fires, for rewarming.

2 PROVIDE WARM DRINKS Soup or high-energy foods, for example, chocolate, will help warm up the victim.

☎ **Call a doctor.** You must always get medical assistance if the victim is elderly, since hypothermia may hide the symptoms of a stroke or heart attack.

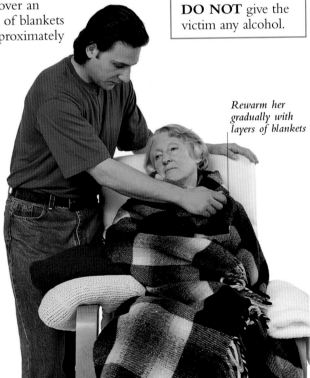

Rewarm her gradually with layers of blankets

STROKE

THIS OCCURS WHEN the blood supply to the brain is suddenly impaired by a clot or ruptured blood vessels. Strokes are more common in later life, especially in those with high blood pressure or a circulatory disorder. The effect of the stroke depends on how much, and which part, of the brain is affected. Major strokes can be fatal, but many people make a complete recovery from minor ones. For an unconscious victim who has suffered a stroke, your main aims are to get urgent medical help and, if needed, begin resuscitation (*see pages 151–52*).

RECOGNITION
There may be:
◆ sudden, severe headache
◆ sudden or gradual loss of consciousness
◆ dribbling mouth and slurred speech
◆ loss of power or movement in limbs
◆ pupils of unequal size
◆ loss of bladder or bowel control
◆ a confused, emotional state

WHAT YOU SHOULD DO

FOR AN UNCONSCIOUS VICTIM

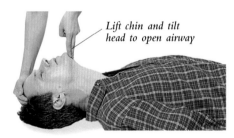

Lift chin and tilt head to open airway

1 **FOLLOW RESUSCITATION PROCEDURE** (*see page 148*) Open the airway, check breathing and circulation. If breathing, place in recovery position.

2 **LOOSEN ANY CLOTHING** Undo anything that may impede breathing.

☎ Call an ambulance. Tell the dispatcher that you suspect a stroke.

3 **MONITOR VICTIM** Check and record the breathing and pulse rate (*see page 161*) until help arrives.

FOR A CONSCIOUS VICTIM

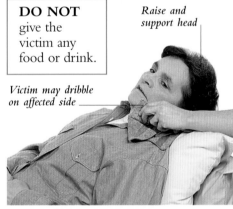

DO NOT give the victim any food or drink.

Raise and support head

Victim may dribble on affected side

1 **LAY THE VICTIM DOWN** Position the victim with her head and shoulders slightly raised and supported.

2 **INCLINE HER HEAD TO ONE SIDE** Place a towel or cloth on her shoulder to absorb any dribbling.

☎ Call an ambulance. Tell the dispatcher that you suspect a stroke.

BROKEN BONES

BONES CAN BE WEAKENED by age or disease, consequently making them more susceptible to breaking or crumbling. Always remember to move elderly people carefully, even if there is no history of violent injury or broken bones. For an open fracture, always stop any severe bleeding first.

RECOGNITION

For a closed fracture there will be:
- bruising and swelling at the fracture site
- severe pain around the injured area

For an open fracture there will be:
- broken skin over the fracture site
- an exposed bone and bleeding

WHAT YOU SHOULD DO

1 **SUPPORT AFFECTED LIMB** Place your hands above and below the injury for support.

DO NOT move the limb unnecessarily.

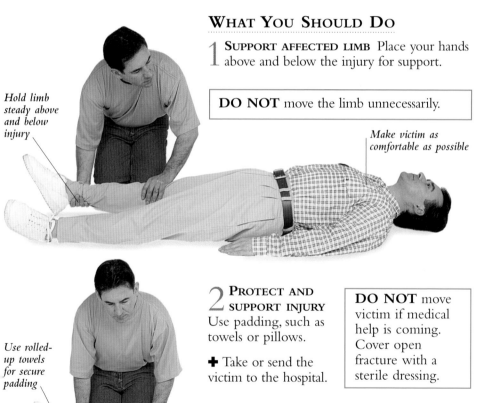

Hold limb steady above and below injury

Make victim as comfortable as possible

2 **PROTECT AND SUPPORT INJURY** Use padding, such as towels or pillows.

✚ Take or send the victim to the hospital.

DO NOT move victim if medical help is coming. Cover open fracture with a sterile dressing.

Use rolled-up towels for secure padding

SHOCK

THIS CONDITION DEVELOPS if the heart fails to pump blood around the circulatory system. It also occurs if blood supply to the vital organs is lost, through severe bleeding or fluid loss. Your aims are to treat any causes of the shock, especially severe bleeding, and ensure that the victim is comfortable. Do not confuse circulatory shock with deep emotional stress.

RECOGNITION
At first there may be: ♦ a rapid pulse, becoming weaker ♦ pale, gray skin, especially inside the lips ♦ sweating and cold, clammy skin **Later there may be:** ♦ nausea and possible vomiting ♦ weakness and giddiness ♦ rapid, shallow breathing ♦ thirst

WHAT YOU SHOULD DO

1 **TREAT ANY CAUSE OF SHOCK** Act quickly to treat any injuries.

2 **POSITION THE VICTIM** Lay her down, preferably on a blanket, but without a pillow. Raise her legs and support them.

Raise legs to improve blood supply to heart

Lay her on her back

Keep head low

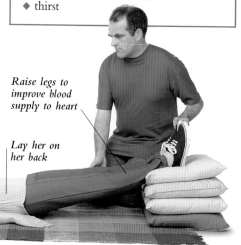

3 **LOOSEN ANY TIGHT CLOTHING**
Undo clothing, such as a belt, tie, or tight collar, that may impede breathing.

> **DO NOT** use direct heat to rewarm.

☎ Call an ambulance.

4 **MONITOR VICTIM** Check and record breathing, pulse rate, and level of response (*see opposite*). Be prepared to resuscitate, if needed (*see pages 151–52*).

Cover her with blanket for warmth

OBSERVATION CHART

ONCE YOU HAVE SUMMONED MEDICAL HELP, it is important to monitor the victim. Make your own copies of the observation chart (*below*) and use one to record your findings, noting the victim's pulse, breathing, and level of response every 10 minutes, or more frequently for a critical victim. The chart should then be given to the medical services, where the information can be used to make decisions about how to treat the victim.

DATE .... **VICTIM'S NAME** ....

		Time (*10-minute intervals*)					
		10	20	30	40	50	60
Eyes Observe for reaction while testing other responses.	Open spontaneously						
	Open to speech						
	Open to painful stimulus						
	No response						
Movement Apply painful stimulus: pinch skin on back of hand, or earlobe.	Obeys commands						
	Responds to painful stimulus						
	No response						
Speech When testing responses, speak clearly and directly, close to victim's ear.	Responds sensibly to questions						
	Seems confused						
	Uses inappropriate words						
	Incomprehensible sounds						
	No response						
Pulse (beats per minute) Take pulse at wrist on conscious victim (*see page 128*); At neck on unconscious victim (*see page 151*). Note rate, if beats are weak (*w*) or strong (*s*), regular (*reg*) or irregular (*irreg*).	111–120						
	101–110						
	91–100						
	81–90						
	71–80						
	61–70						
	Below 60						
Breathing (breaths per minute) Note rate (*see page 128*), and whether breathing is quiet (*q*) or noisy (*n*), easy (*e*) or difficult (*diff*).	41–50						
	31–40						
	21–30						
	11–20						
	Below 10						

FIRST-AID MATERIALS

KEEP ALL YOUR FIRST-AID MATERIALS together in a container and keep the kit in a dry place. Check and replenish it regularly, so that the necessary materials are always available. The types and quantities of dressings and bandages required for a standard kit are shown below, as well as other useful items.

USEFUL DRESSINGS AND BANDAGES

20 assorted adhesive dressings
Use these for minor wounds. The waterproof variety is best for wounds on the hands.

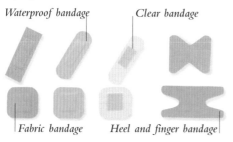

Waterproof bandage   *Clear bandage*

Fabric bandage   *Heel and finger bandage*

6 triangular bandages
These are made of strong paper or cloth. They can be used as bandages, slings, or, if they are sterile and individually wrapped, as dressings.

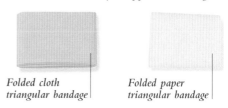

Folded cloth triangular bandage   *Folded paper triangular bandage*

10 sterile dressings
These come in a range of sizes. Ideally, you should keep six medium, two large, and two extra-large dressings.

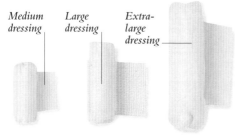

Medium dressing   *Large dressing*   *Extra-large dressing*

2 sterile eye pads
Any injury to the eye needs a sterile covering. Either type shown below will suffice.

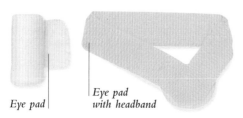

Eye pad   *Eye pad with headband*

OTHER USEFUL ITEMS

In addition to the standard dressings and bandages, the items shown below are useful.

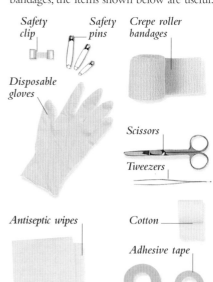

Safety clip   *Safety pins*   *Crepe roller bandages*

Disposable gloves

Scissors

Tweezers

Antiseptic wipes   *Cotton*

Adhesive tape

CHAPTER 15

USEFUL INFORMATION

The pages that follow provide a wide range of
information to help you maximize the benefits and resources
that may be available to you and your relative.

FINANCIAL INFORMATION

The financial section gives details of a range of
benefits to which you and your relative may be entitled. It
explains the procedure for applying for benefits and what
to do if your claim is turned down.

PATIENTS' RIGHTS

The Patient's Bill of Rights was adopted by the American
Hospital Association to protect patients and to make them aware
of their rights to proper medical care and treatment. The
document is summarized here.

USEFUL ADDRESSES

In addition to the help and support provided by your local area
agency on aging, you may benefit from the advice of specialist
organizations. This section gives addresses, telephone numbers,
and other information for a range of organizations that offer
advice and practical and emotional support.

CLAIMING BENEFITS

MANY CAREGIVERS DO NOT CLAIM BENEFITS because they are unsure who to contact or are put off by the application procedure. With a little preparation, however, making a claim should be relatively straightforward. You must be clear about what you require, have as much information regarding your situation as possible, and be patient but persistent.

DO'S & DON'TS

☑ **Do** apply for benefits, even if you are not sure that you qualify.

☑ **Do** seek advice, either directly from the agency involved or from an advice center (*see page 167*), because the system for claiming benefits can be confusing and there are often set rules and procedures to follow.

☒ **Don't** delay in applying. Many benefits are payable only from the date of application and cannot be backdated.

☒ **Don't** be intimidated by the forms or by complicated procedures. Seek advice rather than not bothering to apply.

☒ **Don't** feel ashamed or embarrassed about making a claim. If you do not claim a benefit, you and your relative could lose out on money specifically allocated by the government for the assistance of elderly, sick, or disabled people.

APPLYING FOR BENEFITS

If you or your relative may be entitled to certain benefits, contact the relevant agency by telephoning the toll-free information service or call your local area agency on aging for a referral (*see pages 176–77*). Ask what benefits you could receive and ask them to send you the relevant application forms.

ORGANIZATION TIPS

Try to be prepared and organized (*see box below*).
Obtain advance information Before contacting the benefits agency, find out your rights from a group such as the American Association of Retired Persons (*see page 174*).
Prepare your questions Make a checklist of questions in advance so that you don't forget anything.
Fill in forms carefully Fill forms in as promptly and accurately as possible. Seek advice (*see page 167*) or call the agency for information if anything is unclear.
Keep a record File copies of all correspondence and keep a record of telephone conversations.

INFORMATION FOR A DISABILITY CLAIM

For a thorough assessment to be made, you must supply information about your relative and yourself. Try to prepare some of the information in advance, such as:
◆ Social Security number and proof of age for each person applying for benefits
◆ details of your relative's income and savings
◆ his medical records and results of laboratory tests
◆ a list of all his medications
◆ a copy of his most recent federal tax return
◆ a summary of his work history for the past 15 years

TYPES OF BENEFITS

BENEFITS ARE AVAILABLE from the federal government as well as most state or local governments. Some of the more common benefits are outlined here and on the following pages, together with the criteria needed to qualify. You can obtain further information from pamphlets available from the benefits agencies, or by visiting the local office of the relevant agency.

HEALTH INSURANCE COVERAGE

A variety of health insurance plans are available. Some are free or dependent upon your relative having paid Social Security taxes while employed. Others are purchased by paying an annual or monthly premium. The Medicaid, Medicare, and "Medigap" plans are described briefly below, but you should contact a certified financial planner to make sure that your relative's coverage is adequate and appropriate.

MEDICAID

◆ This health insurance program for low-income people is funded by federal and state governments.
◆ It covers most health care and nursing home costs.
◆ Many physicians and nursing homes accept only a limited number of Medicaid patients because the reimbursement rates are low.

MEDICARE

◆ This program provides health insurance to people at least 65 years old, whether or not they are retired, as well as those with permanent kidney failure or certain other disabilities.
◆ Decisions on claims can be appealed (*see page 167*).
◆ Medicare has two parts. Plan A covers hospital costs, as well as rehabilitation, home health care, and hospice care, and is automatically received at age 65. Plan B, which covers medical insurance, is partly financed by monthly premiums paid by your relative.

"MEDIGAP"

◆ Most people who do not receive their health care through a health maintenance organization (HMO) or managed care program need to purchase private insurance to cover the costs not paid by Medicare.

LOW-INCOME BENEFICIARIES

Your relative may be able to qualify for either of two state-administered programs if his income and assets are limited. Both programs are jointly administered by the Health Care Financing Administration (the federal agency that oversees both Medicaid and Medicare) and the state Medicaid agency.

Specied Low-income Medicare Beneficiary (SLMB) program The monthly premium for the Medicare medical insurance (Plan B) is paid by the state.

Qualified Medicare Beneficiary (QMB) program The state pays the monthly Medicare premiums for Part B, as well as the deductible and the patient's share (usually 20 percent) of any bill. Consequently, your relative does not need to purchase "Medigap" insurance.

SOCIAL SECURITY BENEFITS FOR YOUR RELATIVE

TYPE OF BENEFIT	HOW TO QUALIFY	NOTES
Retirement Benefits	◆ Your relative must be retired from full-time work or be more than 70 years old	◆ Your relative must have paid Social Security taxes while working and have accrued 40 credits or less, depending on age (up to four credits may be earned per year).
Survivor Benefits	◆ Your relative must be the widow, or disabled or minor child, of a deceased benificiary of retirement or disability benefits.	◆ If your relative also receives pensions for work not taxed by Social Security, survivor benefits may be reduced under the government pension offset or the windfall elimination provisions.
Disability Benefits	◆ Your relative must be unable to work and the disability expected to last at least a year or to result in death; or your relative must be the spouse, widow, or minor or disabled child of a recipient of disability benefits.	◆ Social Security Disability Benefits may be reduced if your relative is also eligible for workers' compensation or disability benefits from other programs. ◆ Benefits start six months after disability claim is filed.
Supplemental Security Income (SSI)	◆ Your relative must be blind, disabled, or under 65. ◆ Your relative's income and property value must be below certain limits.	◆ Unlike retirement benefits, SSI depends on financial need, not on having paid taxes. ◆ Benefits may be increased if your relative became blind or disabled before the age of 65.
Black Lung Benefits	◆ Your relative must have been a coal miner. ◆ Your relative must be totally disabled by pneumoconiosis (black lung disease) as a result of working in US coal mines, or the widow, child, divorced wife, parent, brother, or sister of an affected coal miner.	◆ Pneumoconiosis is the only disability for which benefits may be received under this program, and only if it is determined to cause a disability in the individual circumstance. ◆ Claims made after 1974 are handled by the Department of Labor, not the Social Security Administration.

GENERAL BENEFITS

There are a variety of other benefits, available through local governments or charities, for which your relative may be eligible. He may qualify either because he has a low income or because he is unable to work. In some cases, his savings may also be taken into consideration.

GENERAL RELIEF

This benefit, obtained through the Department of Social and Health Services, is restricted to elderly people on a low income who do not qualify for Supplemental Security Income.

INCOME TAXES

There are a variety of tax relief and tax exemption programs that help the elderly. Tax credits for medical expenses (*see also page 45*) and higher personal tax exemptions are two of the most common federal plans. States also give certain forms of tax relief.

RENT CONTROL AND RENT STABILIZATION

If your relative lives in a rented house or apartment, there are many laws that restrict rent increases; in some cases the landlord receives a tax deduction.

VETERANS' BENEFITS AND RAILROAD RETIREMENT BENEFITS

Benefits may be available for veterans or retired railroad workers and their dependents through the Veterans' or Railroad Retirement Administrations.

IF A SOCIAL SECURITY CLAIM IS REJECTED

If the claim is rejected, your relative or the representative payee (*see page 170*) can appeal the decision within 60 days. There are four levels at which an appeal can be made. If the original claim is rejected, a reconsideration can be requested.
If that decision is negative, your relative may request a hearing with an administrative law judge of the Social Service Administration. That decision may be heard at an Appeals Council review. The fourth and final recourse is a civil action in federal district court.

ADVICE CENTERS

The various benefits and your relative's entitlement to each of them can be confusing. There are centers with specially trained staff that advise on a range of issues, including benefits. Among these are:
♦ Social Security Administration
♦ American Bar Association Commission on the Legal Problems of the Elderly
♦ A local senior center
Telephone numbers for these organizations may be listed in your local directory or Yellow Pages; if not, your local town hall or area agency on aging (*see pages 174, 176–77*) should be able to direct you.

Going to a center
Some advice centers have open sessions where you can see an advisor without making an appointment. However, this may involve a long wait. If this is not practical for you, for example, because you cannot leave your relative unattended, ask for a meeting by calling the center or making a request in writing. If you cannot leave your relative alone, it may be possible for a representative to visit you at home.

BENEFITS FOR CAREGIVERS

THE BENEFITS AVAILABLE TO HOME CAREGIVERS are much less extensive than those paid directly to your relative for retirement or health care. Your local area agency on aging (*see pages 176–77*) is the best source of information; many of them have an assistance program to help you with expenses related to your relative's care. You may also be eligible for various tax deductions.

FAMILY CAREGIVER ASSISTANCE PROGRAMS

Most of the local area agencies on aging administer some form of a family caregiver assistance program. These programs are designed to provide relief to caregivers for expenses such as daycare, in-home health services, respite and hospice care, and other services. The funds rarely pay the entire expense of any service; funds are awarded on a needs basis and the amount given depends upon your income.

TAX DEDUCTIONS FOR FAMILY CAREGIVERS

Certain tax deductions and credits may be claimed by family members taking care of an aging, disabled, or sick relative. The following list is a brief outline of such programs, but since tax regulations vary from year to year, your best source of up-to-date information is a certified financial planner or tax accountant, or your local Internal Revenue Service office.
Claiming your relative as a dependent If your relative's annual income is below a certain level and you pay for at least half of his living and medical expenses, you can claim him as a dependent on your federal and state income taxes.

If your relative's expenses are shared by two or more people, one person can claim him as a dependent by filing a "Multiple Support Declaration."
Deducting your relative's medical expenses Even if you cannot claim your relative as a dependent, if you pay his medical bills and at least half of his total support for that year, you can deduct the medical expenses from your income tax.
Tax credits If you work and, as a result, need certain home services or daycare to fill in the gaps when you are unavailable, you may be able to obtain a tax credit for a percentage of those costs.

REAL ESTATE OWNERSHIP

If the person you are caring for is your spouse, you should both be listed as co-owners of any real estate. If your spouse then moves into a nursing home, sole ownership can be transferred to you. This will protect the property for your use and for your relative's heirs, and devalue his assets, thus making him eligible for Medicaid (*see page 165*) sooner. Property can also be transferred to a son, daughter, or anyone else. Like taxation law, Medicaid regulations are subject to change and you should check with an attorney, certified finacial planner, or local Medicaid office for the most current rules.

MANAGING MONEY

Iʜ YOU ARE LOOKING AFTER YOUR RELATIVE, and perhaps other dependents, you may find that you have to balance high expenditures with a low income (especially if you have given up your job). To stay financially stable, you need to minimize your expenditures by working out how you can spend less, and maximize your income, not least by exploring your options for financial help.

BUDGETING EFFICIENTLY

To keep your finances in order, it is advisable to work out a weekly or monthly budget. If you are constantly over budget or short of money for essential items such as food, clothing, and bills, you need to look carefully at your income and expenditures to establish whether you need help.

ASSESSING YOUR INCOME AND EXPENDITURES

Consider the questions below to work out where you could save money or where help may be available.

◆ You may qualify for dependent-care tax exemptions or credits (*see opposite*).

◆ Are you and your relative receiving all possible benefits? Look at the information on pages 164–68 and seek advice, if necessary.

◆ Can you get any help with bills? Utility companies, such as gas and electricity, often have programs for helping people who cannot make a payment. Some charities help people struggling to pay bills.

◆ Are you spending money on items for which you could be receiving subsidies? Some pharmaceutical companies provide prescription medicines free of charge to those who cannot afford to pay for them.

◆ Are you spreading your bills evenly over the year? Smaller monthly bills are often easier to handle than big quarterly demands. Look into setting up a direct debit with your bank or financial institution.

◆ Could others in your household contribute? You may have children living with you who are earning, but don't pay rent. Ask them to contribute, perhaps by taking turns to pay the telephone or food bill.

◆ Is there any part-time work you could do from home? This could just be on a temporary basis until you are more financially stable.

DO'S & DON'TS

If you get into debt, do not panic; there is always a way out if you seek help early enough.

☑ **Do** seek advice. Contact your local area agency on aging (*see pages 176–77*) for a referral that will give you advice on finding a way of repaying your debts. Give details of all your debts, large or small.

☑ **Do** prioritize your debts. For example, it is more essential to pay a utilities bill to prevent the supply from being cut off, than to pay your credit card bill.

☑ **Don't** be embarrassed to ask for help. Advisors will not be judgmental.

☒ **Don't** just ignore the debt. This will not make it go away.

☒ **Don't** take out one loan to pay for another. It may solve the problem temporarily, but it will only plunge you deeper into debt in the end.

GUARDIANS AND CONSERVATORS

If you do not have a Durable Power of Attorney and your relative becomes mentally ill, you will be unable to access money that could be used to pay his bills, or to make medical decisions on his behalf. In this situation, you may need to go to court to have your parent declared incompetant and to be appointed as his guardian. The legal proceedings may be exhausting and, if your relative fights your decision, bitter as well.

If your relative is found mentally incompetant by the court, a guardian is appointed. A guardian may be granted either total or limited authority. A guardian with limited authority may be allowed to handle the relative's personal care, while another person, also known as a conservator, may be appointed to manage financial matters. At regular intervals, both guardians and conservators are required to provide the court with a record of all actions taken and receipts and payments made on behalf of your relative. This protects your relative's affairs and ensures that they are being properly managed.

MANAGING SOMEONE'S FINANCES

You may have to oversee your relative's financial affairs if he is unable to manage them himself. How this is done will depend entirely on his condition – that is, whether he is physically or mentally impaired – and his financial status. You should both seek independent advice from a lawyer or advice center (*see page 167*) before making any arrangements.

REPRESENTATIVE PAYEESHIP AND GUARDIANS

If your relative's only income is Social Security, veteran's, or railroad benefits and he is mentally capable but physically unable to leave his home, apply to the relevant administration for Representative Payeeship. This means that you cash his check on his behalf, while he retains responsibility for filling in claim forms and reporting changes in his circumstances. If your relative is mentally ill, you could become a Guardian. This gives you full responsibility for the account, and for reporting changes in your relative's circumstances. Being a Guardian also means that you are responsible for repaying your relative's debts.

OPENING A JOINT ACCOUNT

This will allow you to withdraw money for your relative's needs whenever they arise. This can be done with accounts in a bank or other financial institution.

ATTORNEY-IN-FACT

Instead of opening a joint account, your relative can designate you an Attorney-in-Fact to operate his financial account and, if he wants, legal and personal matters as well. Your relative must fill out a form in each state in which he owns property.

POWER OF ATTORNEY

A Power of Attorney gives you legal control of your relative's money, but it becomes invalid if your relative becomes mentally ill. A Durable Power of Attorney gives you greater rights over his affairs because it enables you to continue managing your relative's finances even if he becomes mentally ill. However, this right must be granted by your relative before he becomes mentally incompetent.

MAKING A WILL

O NE OF THE MOST ESSENTIAL ARRANGEMENTS to be made by you and your relative is a will. This is a legal document that enables a person to leave his money, property, and possessions to those who are important to him. If a person dies without leaving a will, the law decides how the property should be divided up and this may exclude those for whom he wishes to provide.

MAKING A WILL

It is possible for you and your relative to write a will yourselves but, if it is unclear in any way, there is a risk that your wishes may not be carried out. It is advisable, therefore, to employ a lawyer, who will require you to supply the following information:

◆ a list detailing the value of any property and possessions (the estate), including everything from the amount and location of bank and brokerage accounts, mortgage details, to the value of the silverware

◆ the people (executors) that are appointed to take charge of the estate. This could be a lawyer or accountant (who will charge for the service), but a friend or relative may also be chosen

◆ details of the people or institutions that are to inherit (the beneficiaries), specifying exactly what is to be left and to whom

◆ the value of any debts. Note that a beneficiary will have to repay the debt on mortgaged property unless otherwise specified.

◆ name(s) of any guardian(s) that are appointed to look after children.

TAX IMPLICATIONS AFTER DEATH

Tax exemption If your spouse dies, any property that is transferred directly to you is exempt from estate and inheritance taxes. Ask your local tax office or tax consultant for more information, or request a tax guide at your local library.

Estate and Inheritance Taxes When a person dies his estate is subject to federal Estate Tax if its value is above a certain level. A number of states also have Inheritance Tax, which must be paid by the heir to the state in which the property was located at the time. Even if the person's money and possessions do not amount to a great deal, the value of his property could be enough to make the overall value of the estate subject to various taxes. Foresight and careful wording of a will could save the beneficiaries thousands of dollars.

IF THERE IS NO WILL

If you are dependent on the person you are caring for (for example, he owns the house that you live in) and he has not made a will, you may feel anxious about your future. You can raise the subject tactfully, but you cannot force him to make a will or amend it to include you. It may be that he does not feel ready to make a will because he is unable to accept his impending death; he may see making a will as a sign of giving up, or he may just be too mentally frail to understand. A lawyer or local Citizens Advice Bureau will be able to advise you of your rights.

A Patient's Bill of Rights

IN ORDER FOR YOUR RELATIVE TO OBTAIN the best possible medical care, both of you need to be aware that patients have a role in the decisions that govern treatment choices and other aspects of their care, both in the hospital and after being discharged. All patients must be treated sensitively, regardless of their age, culture, race, language, religion, gender, or physical disabilities.

1 Quality of Care

The patient has the right to considerate and respectful care.

2 Information Regarding Treatment and Medical Team

The patient has the right to, and is encouraged to obtain from physicians and other direct caregivers, relevant and understandable information concerning diagnosis, treatment, and prognosis.

Except in emergencies when the patient lacks decision-making capacity and the need for treatment is urgent, the patient is entitled to the opportunity to discuss and request information related to the specific procedures or treatments, the risks involved, the possible length of recuperation, and the medically reasonable alternatives and their accompanying risks and benefits.

Patients have the right to know the identity of physicians, nurses, and others involved in their care, as well as when those involved are students, residents, or other trainees. The patient also has the right to know the immediate long-term financial implications of treatment choices, insofar as they are known.

3 Patient Choice

The patient has the right to make decisions about the plan of care prior to and during the course of treatment and to refuse a recommended treatment or plan of care to the extent permitted by law and hospital policy and to be informed of the medical consequences of this action. If the patient refuses, he is entitled to other appropriate care and services that the hospital provides or to transfer to another hospital. The hospital should notify patients of any policy that might affect patient choice within the institution.

4 Living Wills and Other Advance Directives

The patient has the right to have an advance directive (a living will, health care proxy, or durable power of attorney) concerning treatment or designating a surrogate decision-maker with the expectation that the hospital will honor the intent of that directive to the extent permitted by law and hospital policy.

Health care institutions must advise patients of their rights under state law and hospital policy to make informed medical choices, ask if the patient has an advance directive, and include that information in patient records. The patient has the right to timely information about hospital policy that may limit its ability to implement fully a legally valid advance directive.

5 Privacy and Confidentiality

The patient has the right to privacy. Discussion, consultation, examination, and treatment should be conducted so as to protect each patient's privacy.

The patient has the right to expect that all records pertaining to his/her care will be treated as confidential by the hospital, except in cases such as suspected abuse and public health hazards when reporting is permitted or required by law. The hospital will emphasize the confidentiality of this information when it is released to other parties entitled to review these records.

6 RIGHT TO INFORMATION

The patient has the right to review the records pertaining to his/her medical care and to have the information explained or interpreted as necessary, except when restricted by law.

7 APPROPRIATE TREATMENT

The patient has the right to expect that, within its capacity and policies, a hospital will make reasonable response to the request of a patient for appropriate and medically indicated care and services. The hospital must provide evaluation, service, and/or referral as indicated by the urgency of the case. When medically appropriate and legally permissible, or when requested by a patient, he/she may be transferred to another facility. The institution to which the patient is to be transferred must first have accepted the patient for transfer. The patient must also be given complete information concerning the need for, risks, benefits, and alternatives to such a transfer.

8 POSSIBLE CONFLICT OF INTEREST

The patient has the right to ask and be informed of the existence of business relationships among the hospital, educational institutions, other health care providers, or payers that may influence the patient's treatment.

9 RESEARCH

The patient has the right to consent or decline to take part in proposed research affecting care and treatment or requiring direct patient involvement, and to have those studies explained prior to consent. A patient who declines to participate is entitled to the most effectivce care that the hospital can otherwise provide.

10 CONTINUITY OF CARE

The patient has the right to expect reasonable continuity of care when appropriate and to be informed by physicians and other caregivers of available and realistic care options when hospital care is no longer appropriate.

11 KNOWLEDGE OF HOSPITAL POLICIES

The patient has the right to be informed of policies and practices that relate to patient care, treatment, and responsibilities, and of any resources for resolving disputes, grievances, and conflicts. The patient has the right to be informed of the hospital's charges for services and available payment methods.

PATIENT RESPONSIBILITIES

Effective care depends upon patients giving information about past medical history, providing an advance directive if desired, and requesting additional information regarding health status if anything is unclear. They must also assist with insurance claims or making other payment arrangements.

Personal health depends not only on the hospital but also on the patient recognizing the impact of lifestyle.

USEFUL ADDRESSES

VOLUNTEER SOCIETIES

American Red Cross
430 17th St. NW
Washington, DC 20006
(202) 737-8300
http://www.redcross.org

B'nai B'rith
1640 Rhode Island Ave., NW
Washington, DC 20036
(202) 857-6600
(202)857-1099 (fax)
e-mail: seniors@bnaibrith.org

Catholic Charities U.S.A.
1731 King St., Ste. 200
Alexandria, VA 22314
(703) 549-1390
(703) 549-1656 (fax)

Volunteers of America
110 South Union St., Ste. 200
Alexandria, VA 22314
(703) 548-2288
(703) 684-1972 (fax)

GENERAL SUPPORT GROUPS

American Assoc. of Retired Persons (AARP)
601 E St., NW
Washington, DC 20049
(800) 424-2277
http://www.aarp.org

Children of Aging Parents
1609 Woodbourne Rd.
Levittown, PA 19057
(215) 945-6900/(800) 227-7294
(215) 945-8720 (fax)
http://www.experts.com

National Assoc. of Area Agencies on Aging
1112 16th St., NW, Ste. 100
Washington, DC 20036

Eldercare Locator
(800) 677-1116
Helps older people and caregivers find local support resources.

Mobility International
PO Box 10767
Eugene, OR 97440

(541) 343-1284
(541) 343-6812 (fax)
Advises on vacations for disabled people and their caregivers.

National Assoc. for Home Care
228 Seventh St., SE
Washington, DC 20003
(202) 547-7424
http://www.nahc.org

National Caregiving Foundation
801 North Pitt St., Ste. 116
Alexandria, VA 22314
(703) 299-9300/(800) 930-1357
Advises on all aspects of caregiving.

National Family Caregivers Assoc.
9621 East Bexhill Drive
Kensington, MD 20845
(301) 942-6430/(800) 896-3650

COUNSELING

American Counseling Assoc.
5999 Stevenson Ave.
Alexandria, VA 22304
(703) 823-9800
http://www.counseling.org
Provides a list of local counselors.

FINANCIAL AND LEGAL ADVICE

American Bar Assoc. Commission on the Legal Problems of the Elderly
740 15th St. NW
Washington, DC 20005
(202) 662-8690
(202) 662-8698 (fax)
www.abanet.org/elderly

Disability in Business Technical Assistance Center
(800) 949-4232

American Health Assistance Foundation
15825 Shady Grove Rd., Ste. 140
Rockville, MD 20850
(301) 948-3244/(800) 437-2423
(301) 258-9454 (fax)
http://www.ahaf.org

Hill-Burton Program
Health Resources and Services Administration
5600 Fishers Lane, Room 7–47
Rockville, MD 20857
(301) 443-5656/(800) 638-0742

Legal Counsel for the Elderly
601 E St. NW
Washington, DC 20049
(202) 434-2120
(202) 434-6464 (fax)

Pension Rights Center
918 16th St., NW
Washington, DC 20006
(202) 296-3776
(202) 833-2472 (fax)
Provides information on pensions and suggests local pension attorneys.

HOSPICE ORGANIZATIONS

Hospice Assoc. of America
228 Seventh St., SE
Washington, DC 20003
(202) 546-4759
(202) 547-3640 (fax)

Hospice Foundation of America
777 17th St., Ste. 401
Miami, FL 33139
(305) 538-9272/(800) 854-3402
http://www.hospicefoundation.org

National Hospice Organization
1901 N. Moore St., Ste. 901
Arlington, VA 22209
(703) 243-5900/(800) 658-8898
e-mail: drsnho@cais.com
http://www.nho.org
Provides information about hospices for terminally ill patients.

ORGANIZATIONS FOR SPECIFIC CONDITIONS
There are many organizations that offer help and advice to sufferers of specific conditions and their families.

AIDS CARE
American Foundation for AIDS Research
(800) 392-6327
733 Third Ave., 12th floor
New York, NY 10017
(212) 682-7440
5900 Wilshire Blvd.
Los Angeles, CA 90036

HIV/AIDS Treatment Information Service
PO Box 6303
Rockville, MD 20849
(800) 448-0440
(301) 738-6616 (fax)
http://www.hivatis.org

ALZHEIMER'S DISEASE
Alzheimer's Assoc.
919 Michigan Ave., Ste. 1000
Chicago, IL 60611
(312) 335-8700/(800) 272-3900
(312) 335-1110 (fax)
http://www.alz.org

ARTHRITIS
Arthritis Foundation
1330 West Peach Tree St.
Atlanta, GA 30309
(404) 872-7100/(800) 283-7800

BLINDNESS/VISUAL IMPAIRMENT
American Foundation for the Blind
11 Penn Plaza, Ste. 300
New York, NY 10001
(212) 502-7600/(800) 232-5463
(212) 502-7777 (fax)

National Center for Vision and Aging
The Lighthouse, Inc.
111 East 59th St.
New York, NY 10022
(212) 821-9200/(800) 334-5497
(212) 821-9707 (fax)
email: info@lighthouse.org

CANCER
American Cancer Society
1599 Clifton Rd.
Atlanta, GA 30329
(404)320-3333/(800) 227-2345
http://www.cancer.org

National Cancer Institute
Building 31, Room 10A07
31 Center Drive MSC 2580
Bethesda, MD 20892
(301) 496-5583/(800) 422-6237
http://www.rex.nci.nih.gov

CEREBRAL PALSY
United Cerebral Palsy
1660 L St., NW, Ste. 700
Washington, DC 20036
(800) 872-5827
http://www.ucpa.org

CYSTIC FIBROSIS
Cystic Fibrosis Foundation
6931 Arlington Rd., Ste. 200
Bethesda, MD 20814
(800) 344-4823
(301) 951-6378 (fax)
http://www.cff.org

DEAFNESS
National Assoc. of the Deaf
814 Thayer Ave.
Silver Spring, MD 20910
(301) 587-1788/-1789 (TTY)
(301) 587-1791 (fax)

Self Help for Hard of Hearing People (SHHH)
7910 Woodmont Ave., Ste. 1200
Bethesda, MD 20814
(301) 657-2248/-2249 (TTY)
(301) 913-9413 (fax)

DIABETES
American Diabetes Assoc.
1660 Duke St.
Alexandria, VA 22314
(703) 549-1500/(800) 232-3472
http://www.diabetes.org

EPILEPSY
Epilepsy Foundation of America
4351 Garden City Drive
Landover, MD 20785
(301) 459-3700/(800) 332-1000
http://www.esa.org

HEART
American Heart Assoc.
7272 Greenville Ave.
Dallas, TX 75231
(214) 373-6300/(800) 242-8721
http://www.amhrt.org

INCONTINENCE
National Assoc. for Continence
PO Box 8310
Spartanburg, SC 29305
(864) 579-7900/(800) 252-3337
(864) 579-7902 (fax)
http://www.nafc.org

LEUKEMIA
Leukemia Society of America
600 Third Ave.
New York, NY 10016
(212) 573-8484/(800) 955-4572
(212) 856-9686 (fax)

MENTAL HEALTH
National Institute of Mental Health
5600 Fishers Lane, Room 1799
Rockville, MD 20857
(301) 443-3673/(800) 421-4211
http://www.nimh.nih.gov

MULTIPLE SCLEROSIS
National Multiple Sclerosis Society
733 Third Ave.
New York, NY 10017
(212) 986-3240/(800) 344-4867
e-mail: nat@nmss.org

PARKINSON'S DISEASE
American Parkinson's Disease Assoc.
1250 Hylan Blvd.
Staten Island, NY 10305
(718) 981-8001/(800) 223-2732
(718) 981-4399 (fax)
http://www.apdaparkinson.com

United Parkinson and Internation Tremor Foundation
833 West Washington Blvd.
Chicago, IL 60607
(312) 733-1893
(312) 664-2344 (fax)

SPEECH-LANGUAGE IMPAIRMENT
American Speech-Language-Hearing Assoc.
10801 Rockville Pike
Rockville, MD 20852
(301) 897-5700/(800) 638-8255

STOMA
United Ostomy Assoc.
19772 MacArthur Blvd., Ste. 200
Irvine, CA 92612
(949) 660-8624/(800) 826-0826
http://www.uoa.org

STROKE
National Institute of Neuro-
logical Disorders and Stroke
Building 31, Room 8A06
31 Center Drive MSC 2540
Bethesda, MD 20892
(301) 496-5751/(800) 352-9424
http://ninds.nih.gov

American Heart Assoc.
7272 Greenville Ave.
Dallas, TX 75231
Stroke Connection
(800) 553-6321

STATE-BY-STATE LIST
OF AREA AGENCIES
ON AGING
Alabama Commission
on Aging
RSA Plaza, Ste. 470
770 Washington Ave.
Montgomery, AL 36130
(334) 242-5743

Alaska Commission on Aging
Div. of Senior Services
Dept. of Administration
PO Box 110209
Juneau, AK 99811
(907) 465-3250

Arizona Aging and Adult
Administration
Dept. of Economic Security
1789 West Jefferson, 2nd floor SW
Phoenix, AZ 85007
(602) 542-4446

Arkansas Div. of Aging and
Adult Services
Dept. of Human Services
PO Box 1437
1417 Donaghey Plaza South
Little Rock, AR 72203
(501) 682-2441

California Dept. of Aging
1600 K St.
Sacramento, CA 95814
(916) 322-5290

Colorado Aging and Adult
Services
Dept. of Human Services
110 16th St., Ste. 200
Denver, CO 80202
(303) 620-4147

Connecticut Community Care
PO Box 2360
43 Enterprize Drive
Bristol, CT 06011
(860) 314-2920

Delaware Dept. of Health and
Social Services
Div. of Services for Aging and
Adults with Physical Disabilities
1901 North DuPont Highway
New Castle, DE 19720
(302) 577-4791

District of Columbia Office
on Aging
441 4th St. NW
Washington, DC 20001
(202) 724-5622

Florida Dept. of Elder Affairs
4040 Esplanade Way,
Bldg. B, Ste. 152
Talahassee, FL 32399
(904) 414-2000

Georgia Div. of Aging Services
Dept. of Human Resources
2 Peachtree St. NW, Ste. 36-385
Atlanta, GA 30303
(404) 657-5258

Hawaii Executive Office
on Aging
250 South Hotel Street, Ste. 109
Honolulu, HI 96813
(808) 586-0100

Idaho Commission on Aging
Room 108, Statehouse
Boise, ID 83720
(208) 334-3833

Illinois Dept. on Aging
421 East Capitol Ave., #100
Springfield, IL 62701
(217) 785-2870
(312) 814-2630 (Chicago)

Indiana Div. of Disability,
Aging, and Rehabilitative
Services

Family and Social
Services Adminsitration/Bureau
of Aging and In-Home Services
402 West Washington St.
Indianapolis, IN 46207
(317) 232-1147

Iowa Dept. of Elder Affairs
200 Tenth St., 3rd floor
Des Moines, IA 50309
(515) 281-4646

Kansas Dept. on Aging
915 SW Harrison
Topeka, KS 66612
(913) 296-4986

Kentucky Div. of
Aging Services
275 East Main St., 5 West
Frankfort, KY 40621
(502) 564-6930

Louisiana Governor's Office of
Elderly Affairs
PO Box 80374
Baton Rouge, LA 70898
(504) 342-7100

Maine Bureau of Elder and
Adult Services
Dept. of Human Services
35 Anthony Ave.
11 State House Station
Augusta, ME 04333
(207) 624-5335

Maryland Office on Aging
State Office Building, Room 1007
301 West Preston St.
Baltimore, MD 21201
(410) 767-1102

Massachusetts Executive Office
of Elder Affairs
One Ashburton Place
Boston, MA 02108
(617) 727-7750

Michigan Office of Services to
the Aging
PO Box 30676
Lansing, MI 48909
(517) 373-8230

Minnesota Board on Aging
444 Lafayette Rd.
St. Paul, MN 55155
(612) 296-2770

**Mississippi Dept. of
Human Services**
Div. of Aging and Adult Services
750 North State St.
Jackson, MS 39202
(601) 359-4925

Missouri Div. of Aging
Dept. of Social Services
PO Box 1337
615 Howerton Court
Jefferson City, MO 65102
(573) 751-3082

Montana Office on Aging
Senior and Longterm Care Div.
PO Box 4210
Helena, MT 59604
(406) 444-5900

**Nebraska Health and Human
Services, Div. on Aging**
PO Box 95044
301 Centennial Mall, South
Lincoln, NE 68509
(402) 471-2306

**Nevada Div. for Aging
Services**
340 North 11th St., Ste. 203
Las Vegas, NV 89101
(702) 486-3545

**New Hampshire Div. of
Elderly and Adult Services**
State Office Park South
115 Pleasant St.
Annex Building #1
Concord, NH 03301
(603) 271-4680

**New Jersey Div. of
Senior Affairs**
Dept. of Health and Senior
Services
PO Box 807
Trenton, NJ 08625
(609) 292-3766/(800) 792-8820

**New Mexico Agency
on Aging**
La Villa Rivera Building
228 East Palace Ave.
Santa Fe, NM 87501
(505) 827-7640

**New York State Office for
the Aging**
2 Empire State Plaza
Albany, NY 12223
(518) 474-5731/(800) 342-9871

North Carolina Div. of Aging
693 Palmer Drive
Raleigh, NC 27626
(919) 733-3983

**North Dakota Dept. of
Human Services**
Aging Services Div.
600 South 2nd St., Ste. 1C
Bismarck, ND 58504
(701) 328-8910

Ohio Dept. of Aging
50 West Broad. St., 9th floor
Columbus, OH 43215
(614) 466-5500

**Oklahoma Services for
the Aging**
Dept. of Human Services
PO Box 25352
Oklahoma City, OK 73125
(405) 521-2281/-2327

**Oregon Senior and Disabled
Services Div.**
500 Summer St. NE
Salem, OR 97310
(503) 945-5811

Pennsylvania Dept. of Aging
Commonwealth of Pennsylvania
400 Market St.
Harrisburg, PA 17101
(717) 783-1550

**Rhode Island Dept. of Elderly
Affairs**
160 Pine St.
Providence, RI 02903
(401) 277-2858

**South Carolina Dept. of Health
and Human Services**
Office on Aging
PO Box 2206
Columbia, SC 29202
(803) 737-7500

**South Dakota Office of Adult
Services and Aging**
700 Governors Drive
Pierre, SD 57501

(605) 773-3656

**Tennessee Commission on
Aging**
Andrew Jackson Bldg., 9th floor
500 Deaderick St.
Nashville, TN 37243
(615) 741-2056

Texas Dept. on Aging
PO Box 12786 Capitol Station
Austin, TX 78711
(512) 424-6840

**Utah Div. of Aging and Adult
Services**
Box 45500
120 North 200 West
Salt Lake City, UT 84145
(801) 538-3910

**Vermont Dept. of Aging and
Disabilities**
103 South Main St.
Waterbury, VT 05671
(802) 241-2400

Virginia Dept. for the Aging
1600 Forest Ave., Ste. 102.
Richmond, VA 23229
(804) 662-9333

**Washington Aging and Adult
Services Administration**
Dept. of Social and Health
Services
PO Box 45600
Olympia, WA 98504
(360) 493-2500

**West Virginia Bureau of Senior
Services**
Holly Grove, Bldg. 10
1900 Washington St.
Charleston, WV 25305
(304) 558-3317

**Wisconsin Bureau of Aging
and Longterm Care Resources**
217 South Hamilton St., Ste. 300
Madison, WI 53703
(608) 266-2536

**Wyoming Dept. of Health
Office on Aging**
139 Hathaway Bldg.
Cheyenne, WY 82002
(307) 777-7986

GLOSSARY OF MEDICAL CONDITIONS

Abscess A collection of pus anywhere in the body. A boil is a common type of abscess.

AIDS (Acquired Immune Deficiency Syndrome). A condition in which the immune system stops functioning properly. It is caused by infection with HIV (human immunodeficiency virus), which is transmitted sexually and through blood.

Alzheimer's disease A name given to forms of dementia (*see* Dementia) not resulting from disease of the brain's blood vessels. It results in loss of memory, confusion, and unpredictable behavior.

Anemia A deficiency of hemoglobin, the red pigment in blood cells that carries oxygen around the body. The most usual cause is lack of iron. Symptoms include pallor and fatigue.

Angina Chest pain caused by narrowing of the blood vessels that supply the heart. When the demand for oxygen is increased, for example during exercise or stress, the affected heart does not receive enough oxygen, which causes pain.

Arthritis Inflammation of the joints. The joints, especially the protective cartilage and capsule, become diseased or worn out, causing varying degrees of pain and disability. Two common types of arthritis are rheumatoid arthritis and osteoarthritis.

Asthma Attacks of wheezing and breathlessness that can become severe. It is caused by narrowing of the airways and is often triggered by an allergy, for example, to pollen or to house dust.

Bronchitis Inflammation of the bronchi, the larger airways of the lungs. Common symptoms are breathlessness, coughing, and production of phlegm. Acute bronchitis is usually short-lived and commonly follows a viral illnes, such as a cold, or inhalation of an irritant substance. Repeated attacks may result in chronic bronchitis, a permanent condition seen especially in smokers and those exposed repeatedly to air pollution.

Cancer A malignant tumor (growth) which, if untreated, can be fatal. Tumors can develop in any organ of the body, interfering with their function and destroying healthy tissue. Tumor cells can travel to other parts of the body to form secondary growths.

Cataract A disorder of the lens of the eye. The lens becomes opaque (milky in appearance), reducing the amount of light entering the eye. It may result in blindness if not surgically removed.

Cerebral palsy Poor coordination and abnormal muscular control of various parts of the body as a result of brain damage, which most commonly takes place at birth.

Chickenpox An illness caused by the virus *herpes zoster*. Often described as a childhood illness, adults can also contract it. Symptoms include a high temperature, headache, and a red rash from which small blisters develop. The blisters are extremely irritating, but if they or their scabs are picked, permanent scarring can result.

Conjunctivitis Inflammation of the conjunctiva, the membrane that covers the front of the eye. It causes redness, itching, and discharge from the eye.

Coronary thrombosis A blood clot in the arteries supplying the heart. It can occur suddenly, usually in arteries narrowed by disease. If the clot fails to dissolve quickly, part of the heart muscle dies, causing a heart attack (*myocardial infarction*). It is accompanied by severe central chest pain (*angina*), sometimes traveling to the neck and left arm, with profound shock and a feeling of doom.

Cystic fibrosis An inherited disorder that is usually present at birth. It affects various glands and is characterized by secretion of sticky mucus, repeated chest infections, and failure to grow properly due to poor digestion of food.

Cystitis An acute inflammation of the bladder. Often caused by an infection, it causes lower abdominal pain together with painful and frequent passing of urine.

Dementia Gradual loss of intellect due to progressive deterioration of the brain cells. It is sometimes the result of deterioration of the brain's blood vessels and is usually, but not always, confined to the elderly. Dementia causes anxiety, memory loss, and confusion.

Depression (depressive illness) An excessive downswing of mood sometimes accompanied by lack of appetite, sleep disturbance, and fatigue. Its seriousness is often under-estimated and medical advice should be sought.

Dermatitis Inflammation of the skin, a variety of which is known as eczema. It results in red, shiny, dry, cracked areas of skin. Scratching causes infection and weeping skin.

Diabetes A condition in which the pancreas secretes insufficient insulin or none at all. Symptoms include excessive thirst, frequent urination, weight loss, and in severe cases, it can lead to coma.

Eczema *See* Dermatitis.

Emphysema A disease of the lungs in which the small air sacs (*alveoli*) are destroyed. It causes breathlessness and can lead to heart failure. Often caused by smoking, emphysema also commonly accompanies chronic bronchitis and severe longterm asthma.

Epilepsy A condition in which periods of abnormal electrical activity in the brain can lead to seizures, loss of consciousness, and possibly convulsions.

Gastroenteritis Inflammation of the stomach and bowel leading to diarrhea and vomiting. It is normally due to a virus or eating contaminated food. Most cases will settle in 24 to 48 hours, but the condition can be more serious if the sufferer is very young or elderly, or if the symptoms are severe or prolonged.

Glaucoma A condition in which pressure builds up in the eyeball. It can lead to permanent damage and blindness.

Hemophilia A hereditary disease that affects males only, in which the blood fails to clot due to a lack of an ingredient known as Factor Eight.

Heart attack *See* Coronary thrombosis.

Hepatitis Inflammation of the liver caused by a viral infection. Hepatitis types A and E are transmitted mostly through drinking water contaminated by infected feces. Hepatitis types B, C and D are transmitted through blood and sexual contact.

Herpes simplex A virus responsible for cold sores and genital herpes. It causes small blisters that erupt on the skin.

Herpes zoster *See* Chickenpox *and* Shingles.

Infectious mononucleosis A viral infection which characteristically results in swelling of the glands in the neck (*lymph nodes*). Other symptoms include high temperature and a sore throat.

Influenza (flu) An acute viral infection. Symptoms include high fever, sweating, and aching muscles. In a healthy adult, the illness runs its course in seven to ten days and a full recovery usually results. Pneumonia is a dangerous complication, occurring more frequently in young children and the elderly.

Laryngitis Inflammation of the larynx (voice box). It results in a sore throat, cough, and a hoarse or lost voice. Laryngitis is commonly associated with infections of the upper and lower respiratory tract, but it can also occur after misuse of the voice.

Leukemia A cancer (*see* Cancer) that affects the white cells in the blood.

Measles A potentially dangerous viral illness, the characteristic symptoms of which are a rash and fever. It is more common in children.

Meningitis A bacterial or viral infection, that causes inflammation of the protective membranes (*meninges*) that surround the brain. Symptoms include severe headaches, sensitivity to light, neck stiffness, nausea, vomiting, confusion, and in some cases, a reddish-purple rash. Bacterial meningitis can be severe and life-threatening.

Motor neuron disease A progressive disease affecting the nerves that control muscular activity. It usually appears in older people and results in increasing disability.

Multiple sclerosis A disease affecting the sheaths that protect particular nerves in the brain and spinal cord. It usually begins in early adulthood and progresses gradually with remissions. It causes weakness, poor coordination, loss of sensation, and eye and bladder disturbances. Mood changes are common.

Mumps A viral illness occurring mainly in children. The characteristic symptom is painful swelling and inflammation of the salivary (*parotid*) glands, located just below the jaw.

Muscular dystrophy A group of hereditary disorders affecting the muscles (but not the nerves). They commonly affect children, causing progressive weakness and consequent deformities.

Osteoporosis A condition in which bone loses its density. When severe, it can cause bending and even fracture of the bones. Hormones have a strong influence on bone density and osteoporosis commonly occurs in women after menopause because production of estrogen has ceased.

Parkinson's disease A disease of the central nervous system. As a result of lack of certain chemical substances in the brain, there is a progressive onset of muscular tremors and rigidity. Characteristic signs include trembling hands, slow speech and a stiff, shuffling walk. It usually occurs in the elderly.

Pneumoconiosis A progressive lung disease mainly affecting miners or construction workers. It is caused by the accumulation of mineral dust, commonly coal (black lung disease) or silica, causing thickening and scarring of the lungs.

Pneumonia An acute infection of the lungs. It is characterized by high fever, shivering, and the production of infected green or yellow phlegm, which may be blood-stained. The infection is usually caused by bacteria.

Polio A viral illness which, in a minority of cases, damages the motor nerves in the spinal cord causing paralysis of a limb or even of the muscles involved in breathing. Vaccination has now virtually eradicated the disease in many countries.

Rheumatism A commonly used term for joint and muscular aches and pains.

Scabies A skin infestation caused by a mite. It is spread by direct skin-to-skin contact. The mite burrows into the skin and causes an allergic reaction with intense irritation. Common sites affected are the finger-webs, wrists, elbows, armpits, the crotch, and buttocks.

Shingles A disease caused by *Herpes zoster,* the virus that causes chickenpox. It affects nerves in the skin and results in a painful, blistering rash. The person is infectious until all blisters have scabbed over.

Sinusitis Inflammation of the sinuses (air-filled cavities around the nose). It is caused by an allergy or an infection, and it may also follow a cold. Symptoms include pain behind the cheeks and the upper jaw. A buildup of fluid occurs that, if infected by bacteria, causes a fever and production of yellow-green mucus.

Spina bifida A defect present at birth in which one or more vertebrae has not developed completely and the spinal cord is exposed. It results in varying degrees of disability. Infection within the spinal canal is the most serious complication.

Stoma An opening in the body that is created surgically. If the voice box is removed, a stoma is made at the front of the neck through which the patient breathes. Stomas are made in the abdomen to collect feces in patients with intestinal diseases.

Stroke Damage to the brain caused by a blood clot or hemorrhage. It can result in loss of consciousness or even coma, loss of speech and other bodily functions, and varying degrees of paralysis of different parts of the body.

Thrombosis A blood clot inside a blood vessel. If the thrombosis occurs in the brain, heart, or lung, the person's life may be at risk. A clot forming in the leg may not be life-threatening in itself, but part of it may break off and travel to the lungs.

Tuberculosis (TB) An infectious, airborne disease that usually affects the lungs, causing coughing, chest pain, and fever.

INDEX

PERSONAL RECORD BOOK

USE THIS SECTION TO RECORD essential information about your relative's special needs, her likes and dislikes, and her daily and weekly routine. Once you have filled it in, it can be used by other people involved in your relative's care, such as volunteers or care professionals. It is designed to be used as a quick reference guide and should not replace a care plan (*see page 33*).

PERSONAL DETAILS

Full name

Date of birth

How he/she likes to be addressed

HOBBIES AND INTERESTS

Reading

Preferred newspaper/magazine/books

Television/radio

Favorite programs

Other interests

COMMUNICATION NEEDS

Impaired speech

Details

Impaired sight

Details

Impaired hearing

Details

COMMUNICATION AIDS	
TYPE OF AID	WHERE IT IS KEPT

EMERGENCY INFORMATION

Relative/friend

Name

Address

☎

Neighbor

Name

Address

☎

Other caregivers

Name

☎

Name

☎

Physician

Name

☎

Registered nurse

Name

☎

Other care professionals

Name

☎

Name

☎

Local hospital

Address

☎

EMERGENCY SERVICES
IN AN EMERGENCY DIAL 911

Address and directions to home

MEDICAL ESSENTIALS	
ITEM	WHERE IT IS KEPT
Medication	
First-aid kit	
Thermometer	

AROUND THE HOUSE

Gas

Shut-off valve

Water

Shut-off valve

Electricity

Fuse box

USEFUL TELEPHONE NUMBERS

Plumber

Name

☎

Electrician

Name

☎

Handyman

Name

☎

Gardener

Name

☎

Essential items

Spare keys are kept

Flashlight is kept

Candles are kept

Telephone

Telephones are situated

Heating

Central heating controls are

OTHER INFORMATION

EATING AND DRINKING

TYPICAL MEALS

Breakfast

_____

_____

Morning snacks

_____

Lunch

_____

_____

Afternoon snacks

_____

_____

Dinner

_____

_____

Bedtime snacks

_____

_____

_____

ASSISTANCE NEEDED

❑ None

❑ Uses aids

❑ Needs to be fed

Other information

_____

_____

DIETARY RESTRICTIONS

Health reasons

_____

_____

Allergies

_____

_____

Likes and dislikes

_____

_____

OTHER INFORMATION

EATING AND DRINKING AIDS	
Fill in special utensils and dishes used	
TYPE OF AID	WHERE IT IS KEPT

PERSONAL CARE

WASHING AND BATHING
☐ No help needed

☐ Uses aids

☐ Needs assistance

Other information

DRESSING
☐ No help needed

☐ Uses aids

☐ Needs assistance

Other information

USING THE TOILET
☐ No help needed

☐ Uses aids

☐ Needs assistance

Other information

MOBILITY
☐ No help needed

☐ Uses aids

☐ Needs assistance

Other information

SPECIAL AIDS TO INCREASE INDEPENDENCE		
Give details of special aids that your relative uses or that help a caregiver to assist.		
TASK	TYPE OF AID	WHERE IT IS KEPT
Washing and bathing		
Using the toilet		
Dressing		
Mobility		

DAILY ROUTINE

NOTE DOWN THE REGULAR TIMES that your relative does certain things, such as eating breakfast or getting dressed, or just prefers to be left alone. Record any routines that a temporary caregiver should be aware of, so that the normal structure of the day is not affected if you are not there. Use the side panel to fill in details of the times that medication is required.

MORNING

MEDICATION TIMES

AFTERNOON

EVENING

BEDTIME ROUTINE

SPECIAL NOTES FOR NIGHT CARE

Fill in details, such as if your relative uses the toilet at night or needs to be turned in bed.

WEEKLY TIME PLANNER

U SE THIS PLANNER TO FILL IN regular weekly events, when your relative attends a day center, for example, or if there are particular days that people visit. In addition to being a useful guide for other caregivers, it can help you plan your own time; use it to note down regular appointments so that your relative is also aware of your plans.

	MORNING	AFTERNOON	EVENING
MONDAY			
TUESDAY			
WEDNESDAY			
THURSDAY			
FRIDAY			
SATURDAY			
SUNDAY			

OTHER INFORMATION

Fill in additional information, such as events that only happen every two weeks or monthly.

ACKNOWLEDGMENTS

The contributors to this edition:
St. John Ambulance
Ann Marie Barnard, Vi Haddow, David
Nobbs, Terry Perkins, Dr. Tom Rogerson,
and Mary Spinks.
St. Andrew's Ambulance Association
Isobel Foster.
British Red Cross
Sir Peter Beale, Mary Coleman, John
Harvey, and Michael Hill.
**Visiting Nurse Associations
of America**
Lex Janiszewski; Interim President, VNAA;
Keith Sessions, Corridor Group

SOCIETIES' ACKNOWLEDGMENTS:
The contributors wish to acknowledge
the advice and help of:
Mary Beecham, Lizzie Lee, Sheila Jackson,
and Marilyn Webb of St. John Ambulance;
Dr. Martin Deahl, Consultant Psychiatrist.,
Hackney Hospital; Olivia Bell, Press
Officer, the Royal National Institute for
the Blind; Maggie Winchcombe, Project
Officer, the Disabled Living Centres
Council; Dr. Donal O'Sullivan, Consultant
in Communicable Disease Control,
Lambeth Lewisham and Southwark Health
Authority; Karen Sorensen, Director of
Dietetics, Guy's and St. Thomas's Hospital
Trust; Barbara White, Customer Services,
British Oxygen Corporation; Dr. David
Woods, General Practitioner, Ely,
Cambridgeshire; Jill Harrison and Gail
Elkington, Carers National Association;
John Bell and Croyden and Keep Able for
loaning aids and equipment; Nancy
Borkstadt; Barbara Pierce, American
Association of Retired Persons; Tom
Humphrey, Children of Aging Parents.

The publishers would like to thank
the following:
For permission to reproduce photographs:
Armitage Shanks, *page 50 right*; Bill Craig
Imaging – Cardiff, *page 93 bottom right*;
Gimson Stairlifts Ltd, *page 47 center right*;
Goldreif, *page 48*; Parker Bath Company, *page
51 bottom center*; Rex Features, *page 5 top left*.
For help with producing the book:
Fergus Collins, Elaine Harries, Maureen
Rissik, Penny Warren, and Nancy
Lieberman for editorial assistance; Sara
Harper, Jennifer Dorr, and Barbara Minton
for proofreading; Hilary Bird for the index;
Carol Oliver, Lucy Parissi, Glenda Tyrrell,
and Anne Redmond for design assistance;
Marianna Sonnenberg, Vicky Wilks, and Dr.
Fiona Payne for picture research; Ian
Merrill and Adam Moore for DTP work;
Robert Farnworth for the illustrations;
Michelle Walker, stylist; Gary Ombler and
Andy Crawford for additional photography;
Andy Komorowski for set building, and
Pebbles for makeup.
For modeling in the photographs:
Georgina Abudulai, Peter Allen, Dawn Bates,
Sue Callister, Margaret Curry, Edward Deeks,
Peter Ellis, Carole Evans, Eric Ferretti,
Mary Ferretti, Yvonne Fisher, James Fraser,
Caroline Fraser Ker, Joany Haig, Elaine
Harries, Lynne Haywood, Stephen Herron,
Clara Inman, Alison Jones, Amanda Kernot,
Ross Mackenzie, Brian Marsh, Nasim Mawji,
Andrew McDonald, Andy Milligan, Hamida
Mohammed, Lucy Parissi, Terry Perkins,
Sigrid Rabiger, Marianne Rainbow, Hoss
Razazan, Simone Richardson, Nick Sarluis,
Alberto Saro, Richard Shellabear, Hugh
Smith, John Walters, Marilyn Webb, Roy
Whillock, Debbie Voller, Pauline Yacoubian,
and Bruno Zeni.